PENGUIN BOOKS

VET IN THE VESTRY

Born in New Cumnock, Ayrshire, in 1926, Alexander Cameron moved to the Maybole region of Ayrshire when his father, a railway stationmaster, received promotion. As a young boy he had a great love of animals, spending all his spare time on farms, and this eventually found expression in his becoming a vet, starting as an assistant in his home area. After two years he moved to Devon, where, in a mixed practice, an added interest was the largest private zoo in Britain. He was a vet for ten years, eventually becoming a senior partner. After great heart-searching, he decided to enter Scotland's Kirk. He studied at Glasgow, where he had also trained to be a vet. His first charge was in his native Ayrshire and from there he moved to one of Scotland's largest churches in Nairnshire. After twelve very busy but happy years, his health had suffered and he was forced to look for something smaller and quieter. He now ministers to four scattered rural charges in the Borders.

Alexander Cameron is married and has four grown-up sons, who all share his love of sport. His hobbies are gardening, fishing and golf. He also has a love of music and has been a church organist.

He has written a number of church histories and historical pamphlets, as well as two plays. *Vet in the Vestry* is his first book.

ALEXANDER CAMERON

Vet in the Vestry

ILLUSTRATED BY JOHN THIRSK

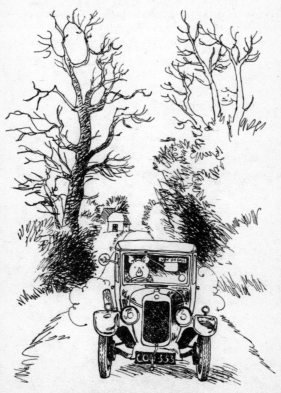

PENGUIN BOOKS

Contents

Preface

Away back in the late fifties, a Scots veterinary surgeon travelled from his practice in Devon to Glasgow for an interview, with the purpose of being accepted for training for the Church of Scotland ministry. It was a hard, indeed reluctant, decision to take, but I felt driven by a constant conviction inside me that this was the way I had to go.

I was interviewed by a bevy of professors and senior ministers with complete courtesy, but also with a sense of amazement, even amusement. Apparently there had never been a former vet in Scotland's Kirk before (though there are at least four now) and the mix seemed a strange one to the committee. I was to find over the years that the general public also thought it unusual, for on hundreds of occasions I have been asked to speak on my two lives, to every conceivable organization. Many kindly suggested that I should write a book about some of my experiences – the interest, the humour, the pathos. So this book was eventually born.

I am very conscious that many will think I am trying to copy James Herriot, whose books have put the work of a vet on the map – and on television – and have given pleasure to millions, including myself. But this is not an effort to 'do a Herriot', for two reasons. First, there is only one James Herriot, and I don't think his work can be equalled. Secondly, eighty per cent of this book was written during convalescence from a lengthy illness years ago, before any of the Herriot books had appeared. It was only recently that I hauled the manuscript out and felt I ought to finish it.

There are bound to be echoes of what another vet has written, for each vet in a general practice treats the same kind of cases, but part of this book is also about my many years as a minister.

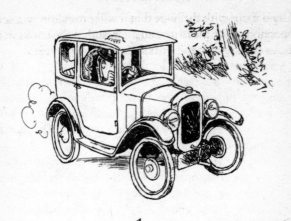

1

The Devil They Know

Andrew warmly shook my hand, helped me off with my gowns, neatly folded them and put them back in their case.

'You'll be the seventh minister I've dressed every Sunday,' he announced. I was startled. I had already realized the general public's idea of a minister was a pretty wet, helpless creature, but I was unaware somebody had to dress him, and looked my surprise. He explained: 'Weel, ye ken, help him on and off with his robes.'

'Hold on,' I said, 'I'm not your minister yet; they've got to vote on it,' a procedure that was at that moment being conducted in the church.

'Ach!' said Andrew, investing the exclamation with such force and vigour that it would counter any argument, 'Ach! Efter that the day there's nae fear.' Then he added, 'You're jist like the gude ministers we've had before.'

I perked up, preened myself, and said that was a compliment indeed, recalling some of the fine men who had

Moderator who was on holiday, said, 'Well, Mr Cameron, after an open vote of the congregation, you'll be glad to know that the vote was unanimously in your favour. May I congratulate you, and wish you every blessing.' Then he gave a smile and added, 'I think this must be nearly unique – a vet in the vestry!'

I thanked him in stammering words; then the committee, led by Duncan the Treasurer, came forward to shake me by the hand or thump me on the back according to their inclination, and one and all to wish me well, in subdued or boisterous fashion.

'Of course,' said one of the committee, 'we never had any doot aboot it, but efter a gude sermon like that the voting was a formality.'

The congratulations over, some of the Elders turned to the important task of counting the offering. 'A gran' collection the day – notes in the plate,' said one.

I thought it time to depart before they passed the plate to me . . . again . . . so took my farewells and headed for my car, case in hand.

'Have you no' a hat?' asked one.

'Never wear one,' I replied. 'I did at one time, but you never saw anything like me in a hat.' Then, realizing I wasn't making much sense, added, 'I just don't seem to suit one, but you might see me in a cap sometimes.'

'Ah, times change,' sighed my questioner. 'I mind when Mr Macdonald came to preach for Moorton before the war, he arrived in a baby Austin wi' top hat an' tails on.' My mind grappled in vain with the picture of a car so attired, till he further enlightened me. 'Mr Macdonald managed to get oot o' the car withoot knocking his hat off, and he was as big a man as you.'

I just grunted 'Good for him,' realizing I would probably hear a good deal about Mr Macdonald in the years to come – a natural thing, for he and the speaker would have been be formally appointed minister of my first charge. Yes, truly it felt good! I was to come to love these kindly folks, and Moorton's storied past. But it was still unreal. What lay ahead, I knew not. Where, if anywhere else, we might be called in the future, I cared not. What was behind me I remembered well.

Three years ago I had been a country vet . . . now I was to be a country minister . . . as brother George had said, it would be a vet in the vestry. But was that any more odd than a doctor, teacher, joiner, farmer, company director, and a host of other occupations which had been represented at Divinity College? I remembered well the short interview I'd had with the selection board before they had decided that, subject to passing entrance exams in the Bible and in Greek, they would accept me.

'Were you really a vet, Mr Cameron? I mean, did you practise?' asked the Chairman. 'Still do,' I replied, at which there had been smiles around the group and a murmur of 'Really!'.

For the life of me I couldn't see anything odd about it. After all, other vets had gone into other Churches. A fellow student had become a priest, and indeed the founder of my Devon practice was now a Canon in the Church of England. But everywhere there had been this same mixture of surprise and amusement, presumably because I was apparently the first of my kind, as far as people knew, in the Church of Scotland. I recalled being rudely interrupted during a Psychology of Religion lecture, in the midst of doodling, suddenly aware that I was being addressed.

'Perhaps, Mr Cameron, you could tell us of your experiences in this field with animals,' suggested the lecturer. Mr Cameron couldn't; I replied to the effect that I had never encountered a neurotic nanny goat or a schizophrenic sow, whereupon my pal Charlie passed along an instant portrait and waxing eloquent about the Canadian prairies, I became aware of a disturbance behind me and discovered a good-going card school in the back seats. So much for my teaching know-how!

I hadn't long to wait, mercifully, for I had a wife and four children to maintain. In a month, the first charge for which I'd applied invited me to be their minister. After ten days' consideration, and feeling rotten about declining the honour these folk had paid me, I had to refuse, for the remoteness of the place was clearly going to present schooling and family problems. I'd applied for another charge in my native Ayrshire, and meantime, with the coming of the summer holidays, I was asked to take pulpit supply in various churches.

I first suspected that I had a visiting committee at an evening service in Kilmarnock. They were there again the next Sunday – and the next. On that third occasion, a glorious summer evening, few of the devout had come to church, no doubt preferring God's good sunshine to the Revised Church Hymnary, second edition, and my elo-quence! But I had a congregation none the less; my visitation committee of four, and, almost at the front of the church, a group of about sixteen, all seated closely together. Obvious-ly another committee – in force. But who were they? I don't know how I preached, nor indeed how I maintained any kind of concentration, for I was highly amused by the glances darting from one committee to the other and the intense scrutiny bestowed on me. I could almost read their thoughts: 'Does he read his prayers?' ... 'Does his voice carry?' ... 'Is he reasonably presentable in appearance?' (I'd heard of one student who was turned down because he had fiery red hair!) ... 'I wonder if he believes in visiting?' ... 'Has he a wife?' – the million-dollar question, this (one of my friends waited a year for a charge largely because he lacked this all-important attribute. Eventually he got a

So I sent in the application for consideration, and left it there. I had no means of knowing whether I would be the selected one in the other short leet.

The following Sunday evening, preaching at Mochrum where I had begun as a young vet years ago, but a long way from Moorton, there was the Moorton committee again; seventeen of them this time, the whole lot. I've no idea how they knew where I was preaching, but the Scot is noted for his 'speirin'', and someone had found out. The service over, I made a leisurely journey homewards, calling at my widowed mother's on the way to spend an hour or two with her. She greeted me with a message that I was to go straight home, since 'a minister and some men' (what ministers were in the human spectrum seemed doubtful!) were awaiting me and would like a word. The minister proved to be the Rev. George, the acting Interim Moderator, and every inch a man . . . the others were two of the Moorton Vacancy Committee. They explained they were from Moorton, had held a meeting that night, and invited me to be their 'sole nominee'. I listened carefully but with an assumed air of nonchalance, as if even St Giles wouldn't tempt me (I was learning fast), and subdued a smile when they, without giving a reason, asked, 'Could you let us have your decision before Tuesday?' Clearly farmers discussed other things at the market besides the price of beasts and the poor pig subsidies!

Janet had been valiantly supplying them with tea and making polite conversation till I arrived, and had withdrawn to let the men – and the minister – talk business. I asked that she should join us in the discussion, because from the beginning our Call had been a joint thing. I protested, I hope sincerely, that they had been less than fair to their other fifty applicants, some of whom were probably friends of mine from Trinity.

'Och, don't worry about that,' said one of the delegation. 'We decided we wanted somebody in his thirties, and we've when he returned from holiday and came to congratulate me, put the ego in its place when he remarked, 'I felt sure Moorton would go for you. You see, a congregation nearly always goes for the devil they know, rather than one they don't.'

That about summed it up!

PART ONE

Mainly the Vet

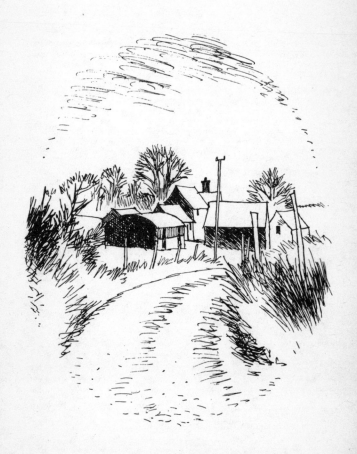

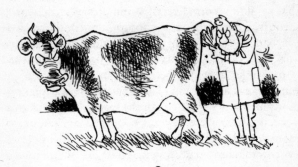

2
The Deep End

I was doing a surprising thing – in fact a daft-like thing. I was sitting at a telephone and longing for it to ring with news of trouble! Here was I, Alexander Cameron, complete with the letters MRCVS after my name, positively God's gift to mankind – or at least to animal-kind, I thought modestly – and the world out there didn't seem to know what it was missing. Nobody needed me! True, in two weeks I would be able to display my talents to the full, for I was then to start work as assistant vet in the little town of Mochrum, where I had completed my schooling, and near where my parents still lived. But that was two weeks away. Today, and for the next fortnight, I was locum for Len Simpson at Glenafton, where I'd been born and had lived till I was fourteen, and where I'd seen most of my practice as a student.

A student . . . my mind went back four days to that scene at the old Vet College in Buccleugh Street, and to the longest hour of my life. We had all just completed our oral finals,

'There they go!' came a shout, and we looked up to see the two external examiners hurry away, to mingled cheers and whistles from about thirty suffering students. We knew now that we had about twenty minutes to wait, because it was decreed that no results be posted till the examiners were safely away – ever since an irate student who'd failed, and didn't think he should have, had assaulted and caused grievous bodily harm to one of the blighters in some past era. Never were more cigarettes consumed, nor such inane chatter uttered, in any twenty minutes since – well, since last year anyway! Some of the suffering throng had been there then, too. You could tell them by the extreme pallor of their cheeks, in thirty faces virtually devoid of colour – except for Bill, who'd had a few too many and was glowing pink. We all knew he'd passed because Bill was brilliant and had gained honours all along the way, and despite the fact that a friend had left him propped against his front door, out cold, the night before the written finals; he'd turned up seeing two exam papers, and had probably passed both with distinction.

But the longest day passes – as some of us had not – and eventually there was a sudden silence as the secretary emerged from the office, sheet of paper in hand, and headed, in a deathly hush, for the notice-board. Then there was an almighty rush, and a series of shouts of relief or groans of agony, as we studied that notice. No names appeared, for we all, like the prisoners we were, had numbers, and there, in an unrepeatable moment of ineffable joy, I had seen number 8 – me! If your number wasn't up – well, your number was up, if you follow me, and you were doomed to more months of suffering. I was quick, but I wasn't quick enough, for others had beaten me to the phones in college and in the surrounding streets. I hared across several Glasgow roads before finding an empty phone-box, and there, all pretence gone now, sent the glad tidings to my mother, forty-five miles

'But *I'm* here!' It sounded a bit pathetic.

'Yes, but you are just a student or something, aren't you, so . . .' Was there anything these country operators didn't know, I wondered? A 'student' or a 'something' indeed.

'I'm not a student . . . I'm a qualified vet . . . I'm Mr Simpson's locum.' In my indignation I must have raised my voice, for back came the 'polite to the public' tone.

'I'm hearing you loud and clear . . . very clearly indeed.' I could picture her holding the earphones away from her head, and probably the whole exchange listening in. 'However, if you just replace your receiver, I'll ring you back.'

'Right-o,' I grunted, and put the thing down.

In a minute it rang. 'Aftonvale 153,' I said hopefully, though forlornly.

'Just testing,' came that wretched female voice. 'The phone seems to be quite all right, Mr Cameron. I expect someone will ring you up eventually.'

She hung up, and I stood gaping. She even knew my name, and that 'eventually' seemed to imply that anybody would have to be pretty desperate to risk me. The wee besom, I thought, probably she had been to school with me – even worse, had been in a lower class. I gnashed my teeth at her condescension, took a few turns round the room, and flung myself down in a chair with the *Veterinary Record*. Flipping through the pages, I came to the 'Wanted' column and read: 'First-year student desires to see general practice, south Scotland preferred.'

That sent the wheels of memory whirling. A few years ago I had been a first-year student about to see my first cases. I recalled coming to this very house all eager anticipation, shiny new wellington boots under one arm, lab coat under the other, and the only two instruments I possessed, a thermometer and a stethoscope, stuffed in a pocket. A long, lean, bronzed individual had answered the door, and hauled me into the room with the warmest of welcomes. I thought

27

The Deep End

It had been just that. A stirk maybe eight months old had been let out on grass for the first time after a long winter indoors. With its fellow Ayrshire stirks at Grassyards Farm, it had run pell-mell about the field, in sheer joy at this new world of freedom. The owner found it collapsed in the field, brought it in and phoned Sandy. From the beginning it was a puzzle, and also a very sick animal. Early on, Sandy had diagnosed a ruptured diaphragm (the sheet of muscle that separates abdomen from chest). It was weird to listen, with my brand-new stethoscope to the stomach, and hear respiratory sounds, and to the chest and hear gastric gurgles. Sandy had suggested he try surgery, but probably to his relief the farmer had declined, and decided 'jist tae leave her alane an' see hoo she'll dae'. We visited her every day for nine days, when – inevitably – she died. A post-mortem discovered a wooden plough handle in the abomasum or fourth stomach. The little stirk had, unknown to the farmer, run full pelt into a single-furrow horse plough sitting in the field, and the force of the impact had snapped off the handle, which had been forced between two ribs – we'd noticed this small wound in the chest but it had seemed of little consequence – and had then gone right through the diaphragm into the stomach. The farmer had missed his plough handle, but hardly expected to find it in a beast's stomach!

That case had been the first of many to illustrate the astonishing durability of bovines, as against almost any other animal. The stomach contents were actually sploshing about in the chest, one lung was completely useless, the other almost so, yet the stirk had lived for nine days! I could remember the quizzical look the examiner gave me when I explained the details. I couldn't blame him. For improbability, it beat any fishing story by a mile.

Two things I recalled about that first 'seeing practice'. One was doing my first pregnancy diagnosis – or rather, he didn't want to know about the work we'd done! Eighteen years old and still starry-eyed with the novelty and excitement of treating animals, I found it inconceivable that he didn't want to know. Sure, it was his honeymoon, but I mean to say, we might be ruining his practice, or stuck and needing his advice! I had yet to learn how completely demanding single-man practice was, and didn't appreciate that this was the first holiday Sandy had enjoyed for years, since the day he'd put up his plate. Yes, a queer phone call that!

Brm, brm . . . brm, brm . . . brm, brm. I sat up with a jerk. The phone was ringing.

'Aftonvale 153,' I almost shouted, in eagerness.

'This is Polquhirter Mains. We've a cow to clean tomorrow.'

'Tomorrow? Oh, I can come out today and clean it.'

'No, tomorrow is the third day. We always leave it till the third day.'

'Sure you're wise?' I queried. 'She's not off her food or anything?'

'Not her! See you tomorrow.'

My hopes were dashed – tomorrow! Polquhirter Mains (pronounced, as any sensible person knows, 'Pa-whirter'): that was Mr Aird. I knew the farm, just half a mile from where we'd lived in Glenafton; in fact we'd bought our eggs there. A cow to clean – that was a nice easy case. I stretched out my arm and rehearsed the job, meticulously removing the afterbirth from the rows of cotyledons, known as 'berries', which stuck out from the wall of the womb in a cow. To remove the placenta was a bit like peeling about fifty little oranges blindfold, the cotyledons varying in size from a hazelnut to a smallish tomato. I shuddered when I recalled the student who'd just pulled the 'berries' off, and the cow had almost bled to death. Oh well, I couldn't get a much easier case for a first, I thought, but decided to check the car

He rushed through his cases to be free for the great expedition of the afternoon, when suddenly, in the car mirror, he spotted the two in the back seat sniggering surreptitiously. He liked a joke, and he asked us to tell him this one. We did, thinking ourselves pretty smart that we'd been able to keep it going so long. The car stopped with a screech of brakes and Sandy went crimson, then a deathly white. He was furious and really tore into us, which we deserved. He demanded to know who had made the call, and his wrath fell on me as I tried to curl up and look insignificant. Suddenly, we saw the thing for what it was: a rotten trick which had gone sour, and caused this man, whom we all respected and who had gone out of his way to help us, a lot of embarrassment. He had apparently rung his bank immediately after the 'garage' had called, and had arranged an overdraft. Students can be exceedingly thoughtless and cruel, and even with the passing of the years, I felt – as I deserved to – very bad indeed about it all. His anger soon passed, but clearly he had been deeply hurt.

So I still felt uneasy, sitting in that room where he had so often sat, and remembering all I owed him. He had even taught me to drive! Sandy was now a vet with the Ministry of Agriculture – a reluctant Ministry man, for he loved general practice. But it had almost cost him his life. Giving a horse a pill, or bolus as it was called – 'balling a horse', to the farmers – his hand had been badly gashed as the horse clamped down on him with its back teeth. He'd given the wound a dab of iodine, and then had gone on for a few days, calving and cleaning cows, lancing abscesses, paring horses' feet – all the day-to-day tasks of the profession. His wound became infected, a raging septicaemia developed, and in hospital, even with the new wonder antibiotics, his life hung by a thread for days, and his convalescence was slow and frustrating for him. His illness had illustrated the vulnerability

He was a quiet man and an excellent farmer, one of the most respected men in the district, a church Elder, and would seldom criticize anybody. He had known of me since I was a wee laddie and must have realized that I was just very recently qualified, but he'd received me with his customary quiet courtesy as if I was some famous consultant who had come to treat his cow, and indeed had apologized for troubling me. Peter the dairyman had joined his boss and me at the cow, and had heard the explanation of the accident. He gave me the whole story.

'It was a young collie I'm training that chased her, the stippit dug. The beast's only a week calved, and just about our best milker. I hope you can dae something, veet.'

I hoped so too, and looked at Mr Barclay with added respect. Most men would have been cursing their dairyman and his dog, but no word of reproach had he uttered. He looked at me now, and said, 'I know it's a bad wound. I can only ask you to do what you can. What will you need?'

I shook myself from the mental paralysis which had seized me, and realized that this man of vast experience was awaiting the orders of a mere novice. At another time I'd have enjoyed this new position of power, but, truth to tell, that ghastly wound had so shaken me that I just wanted to crawl away.

'I'll need lots of hot water, soap and towel, a rope and two strong men.'

'Right,' said Mr Barclay, 'I'll get Bill the ploughman to give us a hand. Peter, leave the milking for now. The cows can wait.'

The dairyman nodded and departed to get the necessities I had listed.

'Bring a halter, too!' I called after him. 'Now, Mr Barclay, let's see where we can cast her – somewhere reasonably clean.'

don't bleed! The flapping skin was first stitched back where it belonged. The hole was a different problem.

'I'm afraid I can't do much about where the teat was, Mr Barclay. I can only try to make the hole smaller, but the pressure of milk will be bound to keep it open.'

I put twenty-two stitches in her, puffed some antiseptic powder over a now dry and reasonably neat wound, gave her a shot of penicillin, and said cheerfully, 'Right, you can take the rope off and let her up now.'

Sixty seconds later my cheerfulness had disappeared, for as the cow lurched to her feet, Peter's dog galloped out from some corner where he'd been lurking. The cow kicked up her heels, broke into a trot, and bang went half my sutures. There was an almighty hullabaloo, shouts from Mr Barclay and his men, and a weary moan from me. It didn't help now that the byreman had caught his dog and was kicking it round the yard. We'd to catch the cow, cast her again, and re-clean and re-stitch the wound. At last it was done – I'd been one and a half hours on my first case.

'Keep her in the byre for a few days, and I'll see her tomorrow . . . and keep that dog out of the way.'

So it was done. The first case was over. As I drove home I reflected that one thing about going in at the deep end was that you had to learn to swim mighty quickly, and were unlikely to be so shocked again.

The next day I cleaned the Polquhirter cow, and as he held the cow's tail the byreman remarked, 'I heard about that job you did at Brockloch yesterday. Sixty stitches, I was tellt!'

I modestly protested that that was a bit of an exaggeration, and marvelled at the speed of the bush telegraph in the country. It appeared that others had heard too, for I was kept quite respectably busy for the next fortnight and the Brockloch cow was a frequent opener of farmers' conversation. It seemed that 'the student or something' had been accepted. The cow did fine and the wound healed without

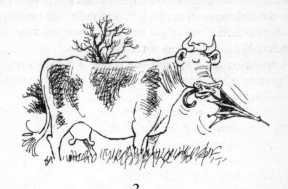

3

Growing Pains

'You'll have to stitch it,' said the boss, holding out a hand encased in a dish-towel which was getting bloodier by the minute. 'We've phoned every blessed doctor in the place and they're all either on holiday or out and can't be reached.' He took the towel off his hand to reveal a badly gashed thumb, blood welling up in it and dripping to the floor, at which sight his wife fled, saying, 'I can't bear to look!' I felt like fleeing after her!

'I couldn't do that.' I quailed at the thought. 'I could drive you to the hospital. It's only ten miles.'

'And sit in Casualty bleeding like a stuck pig for two hours? No fear!'

'But I've done hardly any suturing,' I wailed. 'Besides, eh, er . . .' I paused helplessly, and he grinned and said, 'And I'm your boss so you feel on a hiding to nothing. Come on, Alec, I'm asking a lot, but you can do it.' He plonked himself down in a chair and said, 'Get busy!'

would keep two men fully occupied. Ian Buchan's clients had come to him because he was a good vet, and strong personality that he was, it was not going to be easy for him to trust another with his clients, or for the clients to accept anyone but himself. The position had been made worse by the one assistant he'd had for a few months – my immediate predecessor – who, by all accounts, had been a disaster. 'Pansy', 'cissy', 'dreep', were some of the words I'd heard used to describe him. I'd only met him once and could understand the epithets applied to him. A city-bred lad (which could have been forgiven), with long hair, foppish ways and superior manner, he had, to put it mildly, failed to impress the hard-headed farmers of Ayrshire.

Typical of the stories told me, no doubt by way of warning, concerned Mrs McQueen and her pigs. That worthy woman conducted the young vet round to her piggery, where he gazed vaguely and dreamily into the pen in question, and then took out his comb to sleek back his long hair. Mrs McQueen suggested he might like a mirror, to which he replied, 'Thank you all the same, but I'll manage.' The pigs' owner had then asked him if he knew anything about pigs, and he replied, 'Not much,' whereupon, being a woman of bold speech, sterling character and bulging muscles, she ran him off the farm.

So it appeared I'd succeeded a very bad vet and had come as an assistant to a very good one, certainly where farm animals were concerned. The two facts combined to explain why I had my cases hand-picked for me – that while the boss did eight cases, I was given two, and consequently spent much of my time making up stomach mixtures, scour powders, bloat drenches and the like. When the shelves were groaning with about a year's supply of the various remedies, I was given a supply of Westerns and a comfortable armchair to while away the weary hours. Many boring days I'd put in just sitting in the surgery (which was in fact an anything like this case before? It wasn't calculated to boost one's confidence, and the position was made more difficult by the fact that I'd gone to the local Academy with the sons and daughters of some of them. My parents still lived in the area, and in a little town like Mochrum . . . well, 'a prophet hath no honour in his own country', so what hope was there for a vet?

But bit by bit, with a few cases under the belt on each farm, one came, at least, to be accepted. Mind you, there were many growing-pains to be endured, difficulties to be overcome. Attending a cow at Merkland one day, I diagnosed an impacted rumen (the first of a cow's four stomachs). I knew various stomach drenches would do the job of starting it churning over again, but that Carbachol would be quicker. So I got out my syringe and injected a few cc's into the cow's neck, and closed my case. The farmer continued to glance at me expectantly. Finally he asked, 'Are you no' goin' tae drench her?'

'No need now. That injection will do instead.'

He treated me to a look of withering scorn, and demanded, 'Hoo can a jag in the neck get tae a coo's stomach?'

'Give it twenty-four hours and you'll see,' I said, fingers crossed.

I looked in next day and he greeted me with a huge smile, and took my arm to conduct me up the byre. 'Man,' he said, 'that jag fair did the trick. There's a barrow-load o' dung ahin' 'er. See!' He pointed, and we both stood admiring as if it were gold!

One or two farmers were openly hostile. Many had pedigree herds of Ayrshires' or Aberdeen Angus, most were first-class farmers, and the majority had some knowledge of the various diseases and their treatments; they tended to phone up and ask the vet to come and inject some particular drug, and you had to be mighty sure of yourself if you deviated from their stated orders.

elbows pointing outwards. I gave her a poke just behind the diaphragm and got a decided grunt. The old man, meantime, was alternating between cynical laughter and derisive spitting at my antics. He really was a shocker!

'I'm not sure but there's something more than acetonaemia,' I said.

'And I'm telling you she's stawed! Get the glucose into her!'

'Oh, I'll do that all right, but I'd like to put the cintel on her.' (The cintel was our metal-detector: earphones and a sensitive diaphragm that picked up the presence of any ferrous metal – foreign bodies, as they were termed – which might be lodged in a cow's stomach. At Glenafton we had, in fact, made do with an old wartime mine-detector.) 'I think she's got a wire or nail in her.'

'Damn the fear o' it!' he answered.

'I may be wrong, but I'd like to see what Mr Buchan thinks.'

'Well, see he comes himsel', an' disnae charge me for twae visits.'

The boss was just back from his calving when I walked into the surgery. I told him of old man McNulty and his cow.

'I'll nip up with the cintel after tea,' he said. 'Away you home and get yours and don't worry about either McNulty, father or son.'

So I departed for home, three miles out in the country where my father was stationmaster of two small railway stations. My times off-duty were strictly limited to Friday evenings, and one weekend a month. Otherwise I was on duty at the surgery, or on call, which meant I had to be by a phone. The summons came about eight. 'Rumenotomy at McNulty's; come and give me a hand,' said the boss.

In those days, when straw and hay was held in bales by wire instead of string, and in an area where there were principally wire fences instead of hedges or dykes, a foreign and then, reaching through the incision in the rumen wall, the vet searched about in the reticulum for whatever he could find. The boss nearly always did this part of the proceedings himself, and in this case, after a few moments, he gave a grunt of satisfaction and brought forth a three-inch nail.

'It was through almost right to the head. A few more days and we'd have been too late, Mr McNulty,' he announced, and went on: 'In fact we might still be too late, for that nail may already have set up a pericarditis – that's an inflammation round the heart. But with a bit of luck she'll be all right.'

Old man McNulty was examining the nail feverishly, running it round in his hands, holding it up to the light. In fact he did everything but test it with his teeth. I think he'd have liked to have accused me of planting it, but that being impossible, he rounded on his two workers.

'Damned carelessness, you lazy devils! One of you must have left that lying when you were fencing. If that happens again, I'll have your hides and then it will be doon the road for the pair o' you.' He meant he would sack them, but with his choice of words I had a picture of two skinless men walking down the road, like something horrific from the realms of science fiction. In fact old McNulty was horrific enough, with a face as black as thunder, and the oaths spilling out of him like an overflowing sewer. He was the kind of man who must always have someone to blame.

'Well done, Alec,' said the boss as we headed away. 'I'll charge the old rascal double for doing the operation after hours. He insisted it be done tonight. You should have seen him when the old cintel started buzzing. He nearly had a fit, swore for five minutes, and then demanded that I do something right away. You made a good job of the suturing, by the way.'

I appreciated that. Having got the nail out, he had very

The spike was slowly and solemnly brought forth and handed to Willie, whose large eyes opened another couple of inches while his face fell another foot, making him look more than ever like a sorrowing bloodhound who has just seen his quarry escape up a tree. It was some time before Willie found speech.

'Would you credit that! Nae wonder the beast was no' weel,' he pronounced at last. The boss had meantime turned his face cow-wards and was guddling about in the reticulum, while I discovered I had to bend over the bucket for some time and slowly wash my arms, each thus successfully managing to hide our humour, for Willie's expression would have made the dourest mortal laugh. A piece of wire was found – genuinely – and removed, and the boss could hide his joke no longer, for in truth the situation had become solemn.

'I'm sorry, Willie, we had you on. There was just the wire,' he said.

It was some time before this dawned on Willie, who was still gazing awestruck at the spike. 'So it wisna' this at a'?' he finally managed.

'No, Willie, it was the wire,' said the boss, 'and though I'm not certain, I think, Willie, that's just a bit of it, and there's another bit already broken off in her chest. Keep your fingers crossed.'

Stories should have happy endings, as most authors would agree, but in real life it is not always so. In this instance old McNulty's cow survived, while likeable, friendly Willie's beast died a few days later; which maybe supports the old Scots maxim that 'the de'il's kind to his ain'!

byre?' he asked. I nodded. 'I was out there at a milk fever this morning and as we were coming out the door he stopped and pointed up at a beam in the roof. "Do you see that?" says he. "Do you think I could reach it?" "Never," says I. "Oh well, I reached it last nicht," he told me.

'Seemingly he and his dairyman had just come out to start the evening milking, when the bull came at them. He'd broken his chain, and you know he's a treacherous brute. Well, they both turned and ran for the door; the dairyman got there first and slammed it behind him. So, with the bull breathing down his neck, MacFarlane jumped, caught the beam, and sat there looking down at his bull glaring up at him and pawing the floor. Eventually MacFarlane walked along the rest of the beams which go on into the next byre and got out the door there. It was some jump, Alec. It's amazing what you can do with a bull at your back.'

He paused, lit his pipe, then went on. 'I mind when I was blood-testing the herd at Dalwhinnie – I don't think you've been there yet – but the couple there have a wee boy who's a mongol child. They've also got a notorious bull. The wee fellow didn't like me "jaggin' his coos", so he walked away saying, "I'll get somebody that'll sort you." He did too, for he came back leading this big brute with a piece of binder cord through its ring. He led him right up the byre to me and said, "There he's, Jock – get him." I looked round for the farmer, and he was already up on the milk pipe out the road.'

'What did you do?' I asked.

'Stayed put where I was, between two cows where the bull couldn't get at me. The farmer spoke quietly to his boy – but still hanging on to the milk pipe, mind you – and at last the boy went away, and that bull followed him like a pup on a lead.'

'How do you account for something like that?'

'I don't know, Alec, but I think it's just that these kids don't know any fear, and the animal senses it. Take Spike' the buildings shouting: 'Hello! Anybody about?' I couldn't find a soul, so went looking for the patient and came to a pen with a sow and seven piglets. 'Aha,' I reasoned, having 'O'-level maths, 'I bet the patient's the one that makes eight. It will be lying in the house.' It was a typical pig-pen with a concrete exercising yard and feeding trough, and the pig-house built on to it with a low door for the pigs to get out and in. There was another door round the back, but it seemed to be all blocked up; so I jumped into the pen and crawled through the wee low door, my black case in my hand. Sure enough, there lying on the straw was a piglet. He wasn't all that sick, for as soon as I'd inserted the thermo-meter into his rectum he hollered loudly, there was a great snort from outside, and in came mother at the trot, mouth open, heading straight for me. She had a fine set of teeth, and she evidently meant to use them. I leapt to my feet as she took a snap at my leg. She missed, but only just, and got a mouthful of corduroy trousers. She stood looking at me, as much as to say: 'The corduroy is just for starters, now the main course,' while I eyed her, fending her off with my case.

I licked my lips and glanced around nervously. The proper door was blocked up with bales of straw, and I wasn't going to turn my back on that wild beast to remove them. I sort of sidled along the wall towards the low door I'd come in. The sow sidled along too. It was stalemate, and for some time we just stood and watched each other, neither of us liking what we saw. When I thought her eyes wavered just a fraction from me towards her offspring, I made a sudden dive for that door and crawled through it. No rabbit ever dis-appeared down its burrow quicker than I exited from that pig-house. I didn't stop to look behind me, but with coat-tails flapping and black case bursting open, I leapt the wall. I just made it too, as she came after me for another tasty bite. Evidently the first taste of my trouser leg had whetted her appetite. I was vaguely aware of a figure standing before me

53

one was, I usually got somebody to push the beast's tail straight up or have its nose held, both traditional means of restraint. Today I just boldly went forward, flutter-valve on the sulphamezathine bottle at the ready, and stuck the needle into the vein. The next moment I was flat on my back in the middle of the byre. I'd never even seen the foot come up, but I sure felt it. Getting kicked by cows, or having one's toes trodden on, was an almost daily occurrence, but that was the father and mother of all kicks. She looked round to see the effect of her nifty back-heeler, then went on chewing the cud, satisfied she'd done a good job and had given, in the old man's absence, a typical McNulty welcome. I searched round the byre for some time before I found the needle, shuddering to think what the old boy would say if a further rumenotomy disclosed a hypodermic needle. Taking a clean one from the box, I injected the drug subcutaneously behind her shoulder, a safe position half-way between horns and hind legs. I didn't know whether the drug was effective this way, since it had always been given straight into the bloodstream before, to hit the bug hard and produce a knock-out blow, emulating the cow's style! Apparently it did work, so that was one fact I'd learnt, and – more important – never again to attack the mammary vein of a fit, unrestrained cow.

What with the risk of contracting brucellosis, anthrax, rabies, psittacosis, mange, tapeworms and a host of other cheerful things, I was finding that my profession was somewhat hazardous. But it was fascinating too, and as I bumped along the side-roads of my native county I was learning all the time and was content with my lot. I was even learning how to handle the car I'd been given. It was an ancient Standard whose back springs were gone, so that cornering produced a decided tilt, a horrible rubbing sound and the smell of tortured rubber. In fact, it was not unlike the motion of a ship, and to add to the nautical illusion there was a regular splash of water. Just above my head was a hole ficiently to allow him to swerve on to the footpath and nip out in front of the bus, to the astonishment of passengers and driver. Yes, in those days before MOT tests for a car's roadworthiness, there were as many dangers to the budding vet just driving to the farm as awaited him when he arrived. I suppose it all came into the category of learning to be vets.

The days were full of interest and incident, with new cases and the occasional new client. Came the day when I gained one. Mrs Buchan came through from the telephone looking extremely worried, and not for the first time I realized what a strain was imposed on the wife in a practice which could not afford a receptionist/secretary. It seemed that Mr Wallace had a cow which had choked on a potato and was badly swollen with the build-up of gas. He had phoned for his own vet who was miles away and unable to be contacted, as was Mr Buchan. Now, Mr Wallace was an important man in the area, being an employer of many men, but he also farmed. So I could understand Mrs Buchan's anxiety when she asked me if I could come out, and if I knew what to do. I knew all right, but didn't tell her I'd never seen, far less treated, a choke before. However, after throwing a probang, trocar and cannula into the car, I hurried at the Standard's full rate of knots to the farm. I was received somewhat suspiciously by Mr Wallace himself. He was used to experienced vets, and I could read the doubt in his glance as to whether this young fellow knew what he was about. The case was fairly desperate; the cow was badly bloated and on the point of collapse. I got the long probang over the beast's throat and gave the potato a few taps, but it was stuck fast, and the animal was ballooning by the minute to bursting-point.

'I'll have to stick her,' I said.

'I think you will,' he agreed.

So, recalling from our college lectures how to work out the spot for stabbing the rumen, I tried, and only then realized how tough a cow's hide could be. I couldn't get the would be sundry explosions coming from her rear, and by morning, a good load of dung.

The weeks and months sped past, full of interest now. Except on that precious Friday evening off, it was strictly duty. However, if there was nothing pressing I could stay at home in the evening and have any calls relayed. But one day the boss decided it would be a considerable asset to have a few kennels in a small brick building at the top of his garden, so for some time there were few evenings off. I'd never been a bricklayer or plasterer before, but the kennels shot up in no time – it's amazing how quickly you can work just in order to keep warm! With two of us working, and with only a small number of kennels, the boss was able to encourage the small-animal side of practice, something he'd wanted to do for a few years. An evening consulting hour was started, the first boarders arrived, and dogs could be kept for a couple of days after whatever surgery they had undergone. Small-animal operations were always done in the evenings; sometimes it being ten o'clock before we were able to start. The boss initially did all the surgery; I was anaesthetist and general factotum. I thought him a good surgeon, and certainly he was with farm animals. Comparing him with Kenneth later, Ian was not in the same class in the field of small animals – but in relation to both of them, I was a complete dud. My fingers were all thumbs, and my general surgical technique left a lot to be desired.

I recall the evening when the boss told me to spay a cat, and he would assist. A simpler operation can hardly be imagined, and I'd seen him do a fair number. With my patient safely anaesthetized, I made my incision, and poked about looking for ovaries and uterus. I kept finding loops of small intestine, but no uterus. I looked at the cat again to make sure it was a female, then enlarged my incision and groped and guddled some more. Finally, with sweat blinding me, I said to the boss with what dignity I could muster, 'I dog through the day Mrs Buchan would sometimes put it in a kennel till one of us came in. This particular morning I arrived, and was told there was a labrador in kennels, to be destroyed. For some reason, the boss liked to use a humane killer for large dogs. The gun was one of the captive bolt type and I hated it, but an assistant has to do as he's told, so I went into the kennels with the humane killer, brought out a handsome-looking labrador, held him firmly by the collar, put the weapon to his head, and pulled the trigger. At the very last moment he jerked his head, let out a howl as the gun went off – then he was off, and I was left with his collar in one hand and a smoking gun in the other. I'd forgotten to make sure the outer door was properly closed, and he was out, down the drive and away. It was horrific, for I knew the bolt had broken the skin and drawn blood. As white as a ghost, I'm certain, I ran after him, weapon still in one hand, collar in the other. He was headed for the town, and had anyone been about, very likely they would at once have phoned the police or the nearest lunatic asylum, with a wild-looking man charging about the place with a gun. Fortunately there was not a soul on the street; equally fortunately, I had been told the dog's name was Rex, so hollering 'Rex . . . Rex . . . Here, boy' I kept going and, miracle of miracles, he eventually stopped at the sound of his name. I slipped the collar back on him, tried not to look at this poor beast with a small hole in his skull spurting blood, then took him back to kennels, shut the door and finished the job. I had to grit my teeth to do it, and felt the biggest rotter in creation. That trusting dog had stopped at the sound of his name, let me lead him back to a place of terror – and there I'd betrayed his trust. Ugh! I must have looked pretty ghastly when I went in the surgery door, for Mrs Buchan asked me what was wrong, and I told her the tale. She also said 'Ugh!', then poured a strong cup of tea. Later in the day, the boss cornered me.

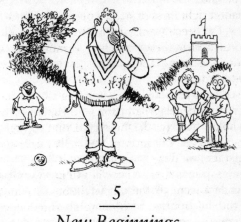

5

New Beginnings

'Mr Cameron,' a lass said to me the other day, 'Brian and I are getting engaged a year come the first of June, on my birthday.'

I had a quiet smile to myself at her earnestness, but when she had gone, I sat at my desk and thought back over the years. That girl seemed part of the modern way: you fix your engagement in advance. It seems so matter-of-fact, so staid, so planned, so apparently lacking in romance.

My mind went back over the years to a bright summer day in June. Janet and I had gone to the Heads of Ayr for a swim, a picnic, an afternoon away from the grind of veterinary practice and teaching maths. On the way back up over the hill to the car, as I watched her swinging on ahead of me, I suddenly realized I could not live without this girl any longer, and there and then asked her to marry me. Her eyes sparkled, she drew a great, deep breath, a smile seemed to engulf her whole being, and she said, 'Oh yes!'

own dream world, walking on a pink cloud, looking in furniture shops and deciding what we would have in our own home. (Some of the articles we haven't got yet!) The sun often shines on the Ayrshire coast, but never did it shine more brightly from a magically blue sky as on that glorious day. One week later we bought the ring and all was official. My father thought we were rushing things . . . after seven years! But he was fond of Janet, as was my mother, and they gave their blessing. In a state of extreme trepidation, I approached Mr Morrison and asked for leave to marry his daughter, and to my profound relief he raised no objections. I left with my legs trembling, but my heart singing.

Now something had to be done about the future. I was not overpaid at Mochrum at £10 a week, and although Ian Buchan dropped occasional hints about a future partnership, there was nothing concrete. More important, much as I respected him I felt I could not happily work in partnership with him for the rest of my life. I would always be very much the junior; and, having had a Church upbringing, and at the considerable risk of seeming 'holier than thou', I felt that if I was going to enter into a *life* partnership it should be, if possible, with a more kindred spirit.

So I advertised in the *Veterinary Record*, and – wonder of wonders – in a few days came an offer to come to Bristacombe and discuss a possible partnership there. It was March, one of the busiest months in the vet's year, but Ian gave me a weekend off and, none more Scottish than a Cameron, I set off by train for the foreign land of England. I was met at Bristacombe station by an enormous individual and a very small one – Major Kenneth Davidson and a student, Tom Atkins.

We had a short drive to Chade Lodge, I was shown to my bedroom, and then, to my utter surprise and some embarrassment, this strange new acquaintance dropped to his knees and prayed that we would be guided as to our future.

phone calls needed an interpreter as I could not understand the Devonian dialect, and the Devon farmers found my Scots tongue equally bewildering. The farmers' names for diseases were different from those used in Ayrshire, and every bovine seemed to be 'he', whether male, female or neuter. I remember holding the telephone away from my ear in total astonishment when asked to go and see 'a bullock bad to calve'.

I learned much in those early months, just watching Kenneth at work, for he was a fine vet, a good diagnostician and a magnificent surgeon, beside whom I was a bungling amateur. I also learned that his faith was the mainspring of his life, and while some of his clients pulled his leg and others shared his beliefs, all respected him. Every day before afternoon surgery we would meet, compare notes on cases, read a few verses of the Bible and have a short prayer. In time my embarrassment and awkwardness gave place to a very real admiration, and some of the naturalness of Kenneth's faith became mine. He tried to run his practice as a genuinely Christian concern, right down to the moderate charges for the new, wonder antibiotics for which many vets, having a monopoly of them, were charging extortionate prices. We were very different in personality and background – he was a colonial, born in Kenya, the product of a public school, a former major in the Indian Army, a man of substance, a big man in every way – while I had grown up in a council house, gone to the local school, and was as ordinary as it is possible to be. Yet we were one, bound together by a common bond, not just as vets but as brother Christians.

My brother Fergus came down to Bristacombe to share the long drive north for the wedding, in those days before there were any motorways. A few days later, on 15 August, with two bridesmaids and my twin brothers Graham and Fergus as groomsmen, Janet and I were married in the little get on with the job as if I had been as experienced as he was. The practice was still at the growing stage, far too much work for one but barely enough for two, so, building for the future, I at first took just £6 a week from the takings and we lived on Janet's salary. Kenneth and I had great dreams of branch practices and expansion, and we were sure we would grow. This indeed happened; we soon opened two branch surgeries, but neither of us saw the final fruits of a veterinary hospital – five vets working together and several lay staff and nurses. We worked very hard indeed, and the seed was sown for future growth.

Right from the beginning, Kenneth tried to involve me in the life of his Church, the Church of England. So I taught in the Covenanters, a youth movement which was a Bible class for older teenagers on a Sunday, and a youth club through the week. My initiation into the first club night produced some pain and not a little mirth. It was a cricket night, and I was fielding at mid-on to the smallest boy in the club. He gently hit a ball in my direction, I got down on my knees to casually gather it, and at the last minute it bounced and hit me a whack on the nose, to the delight of the youngsters and the embarrassment of the new leader. Some fielder! I had a swollen nose for a time afterwards, which did not look too good on a newly married man!

As far as teaching was concerned, I was a novice. I had once, when I was a serious sixteen-year-old, taken the tiny tots in the Sunday School at Maryshall when my father couldn't be there. I took the task very seriously, prepared a talk on 'The love of God', and by way of illustration explained to the children, 'You know your mummy loves your daddy – they love you – you love your brothers and sisters, I hope; well, God loves you like that.'

That's right, Mr Cameron' (Mr! I'd never been addressed like that before), 'my mummy does love my daddy. She sits on his knee!'

practice, and who still works away in glorious North Devon. That is, though, a leap forward in the sequence of this story, so let me get back in line. I owe much to Kenneth, more than I can ever express, and likewise to Bernard, who, though he was a totally different character – quiet, un-assuming – but with the same sure faith, took Kenneth's place in every way. I don't believe I ever expressed my thanks to them and my indebtedness to them both, but perhaps if they ever read this they will accept a belated thank-you for our marvellous years together.

By the spring of the year after our marriage, it was clear a baby was on the way. We prepared for its coming with all the joy and anticipation of every young couple. Janet was sometimes far from well . . . indeed had a rough time in pregnancy, but she was as uncomplaining as she has always been and buoyed up with the thought of the new life that was at the end of it all. Two days after our wedding anniversary, on 17 August, I ran her to the local maternity hospital and left her there; it was quite out of the question in those days for a father to be present at the birth, even though he was a vet who had delivered many young things and was not likely to faint at a childbirth. I returned from my visits – I had flown round in my excitement – to be met by a very agitated Kenneth, who told me the doctor wanted to see me. With sinking heart I visited the doctor, not knowing what his news would be, but certain it must be bad. The doctor was uneasy, and I've felt to this day he had a right to be uneasy. The baby had been stillborn, which of course still happens from time to time, despite our many advances. But the doctor had allowed Janet to go three weeks over her time, the baby was very large for a first, its heart had been beating fifteen minutes before the birth, but it had been lost in the delivery.

We mourned for our little babe, and comforted one

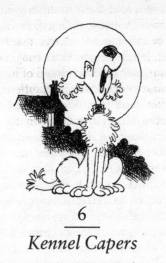

6

Kennel Capers

'Ow--ooo----ooooo! Ow---ooooo--ooo---oo! Ow---ooo –
Wow-wow-wow-ooooooooah!'

Thud! My feet hit the bedroom floor.

Bang! An upstairs window was flung open.

'Shut up, you noisy dog, or you'll be sorry!' – my dulcet
tones floated over Chade Valley. This was the ritual almost
nightly now in our lives. Gone were the days of tranquillity
in that delightful little flat at Langleigh Farm, where Janet
and I began our married life. The farm was just on the fringe
of the town, nestling at the foot of the mighty Torrs, and
sheltered as it was in its ring of trees it was a perfect haven of
peace, a delight to come home to when the day's work was
done and where no hideous cries disturbed the hush and
stillness of night. The only sounds were the bleating of sheep
grazing the Torrs, or the contented cluck of hens as they
strolled about the yard. Periodically farmer Conibear's
voice would be raised as he called directions to his dog

railway station, there to be linked to their great long line of coaches. Below us, at the foot of the steep-sided valley, was the little township of Chade, composed of new council houses and much older terraced dwellings, but now part of Bristacombe itself. So our days were made hideous by sudden explosions of escaping steam from the monsters above us, though in truth they were magnificent dinosaurs, and over the years we would get grins and waves from the engine driver and his fireman, who could look right into our bedroom windows.

Night brought a cessation of steam explosions, and it was then that some horrible canine, thinking that things had gone a bit quiet, would decide to bay at the moon or recite poetry to his fellow inmates, and rouse us and the dwellers in the valley below – seemingly on the principle that if you couldn't sleep, it was much cheerier to have someone awake with you. So nightly, as Kenneth had done before me, I bellowed at the brutes! He had early made the discovery, later seconded by me, that while a tone of sweet reasonableness was maybe all right for a dog in its home, it availed nothing with a howling hound in kennels. You simply had to shout louder than it. Generally the bloodcurdling threats I uttered had the desired effect as the beast got the message. But the crafty ones would wait till you were nicely tucked up in bed again, about to drop off – and then recommence their nightly song, with others readily joining in the chorus. Then feet had to be shoved into slippers, a dressing-gown or coat thrown on, and with set face and fixed purpose I would have to enter the dark kennels, locate the culprit if possible – not always easy, for very quickly they could look like a class of innocent children when the teacher whirls round to spot the offender. If located, he or she heard my threats uttered at close range; if unlocated, they were all bawled out. If verbal reasoning failed, then one had to try manual persuasion, that terrible thing corporal punishment, now regarded as a and 'gone away', making it a trifle awkward when the owner returned. When the mantle of night fell on the scene, the responsibility for keeping the peace was mine. Such was the vehemence with which I verbally assaulted these dogs, daily threatening to come and knock their blocks off, murder them, or generally cause life to be unpleasant for them, that I was sure I heard the words 'Shut up!' from our infant son in almost his first coherent utterance. This indeed was a sobering thought. Suppose he used the phrase to either of his grandparents, or treated the minister to his party piece? I can only hope that I was mistaken, for I'm certain that psychologists would unanimously declare that I had caused irreparable damage to a child's mind. Be that as it may, what is certain is that from a very early age he would sit in his high chair, and when the dogs were giving tongue in their premises would point an accusing finger in their direction and sternly order, 'Quiet, wow-wows!'

But we kept more than dogs at our kennels. In a steeply sloping one-acre field which ran parallel with the drive up to Chade Lodge resided Susan and Veronica, respectively Large White and black-and-white Wessex Saddleback sows. I was already well acquainted with them before we moved into the Lodge. Kenneth had his very new Triumph saloon, while yours truly had the antiquated van initially, so when either Susan or Veronica expressed a wish to visit their mutual husband who dwelt on a farm just outside the town, there was only one vehicle that could be used to transport them. From time to time S. or V., or occasionally S. and V. together, would be coaxed, cajoled and generally heaved into COD 330's interior, something that long-suffering vehicle had experienced many times before as it had often carried pigs of both sexes and all ages and sizes (albeit never the live kind, having in fact formerly been a butcher's van). I will always remember those hair-raising trips with pigs as my companions. No partition separated the driver from the

'Hey, mister,' announced our visitor, 'there's some little pigs running about on the main road!'

'How many?' I asked – a daft question, as if it mattered, but I'm not at my brightest, un-breakfasted. The spokesman said three, but his attendants quickly corrected him, in numbers varying, as far as I could make out, from one to thirteen. Clearly something had to be done about it, so accompanied by my self-appointed assistants I hurried down the field to the scene of action – readily spotted, since the rest of the gang were all there before me. In a couple of minutes all became clear, though it was to take much longer to correct the situation.

What had happened was that sometime during the night Veronica had felt her time had come to produce another litter. I suspect that she was turfed out of their house by Susan, always the boss, and probably in one of her moods. Now, the field was very steeply sloping indeed, and apparently the only reasonably level, sheltered and seemingly private bed Veronica could find was right under the hedge, which grew, Devon-style, on top of a wall, some ten feet above the main Chade–Bristacombe highway below. There she had given birth, and continued to do so, producing at regular intervals another little black-and-white minstrel. Since sows frequently take some time to deliver the complete litter, clearly the early arrivals felt they couldn't hang about for ever to see how many brothers or sisters they would have but had set about the immediate task of finding food, readily available from any one of the teats neatly arranged on Veronica's undercarriage for that very purpose. The trouble was that with her feet sticking through the hedge, it became a hazardous journey for the newly-born to find the feed trough! The easy way was to walk over mother, but on that already steep gradient her side acted as a shute, propelling her offspring out into the unexplored depths below, where they hung about waiting for something to

79

proceeded to do – disappear fast – before the Cruelty man, the police, the fire brigade or any other body was summoned to the scene. The van was hastily driven down the road, and, assisted by dozens of children having the time of their lives, I tried to round up the now scattered minstrel chorus and pop them in the van. The two remaining 'barnacles' were removed and pushed in front of Veronica's snout; and my poor wife, using these two as bait, proceeded to shoo the lady of the moment to her shed, where she was reunited with her offspring, or most of them. For all I know, some family in the Chade housing estate had roast sucking pig for supper that night, but we still had a fair number, and Veronica seemed well content with her brood and with a job well done. That was the last straw. I felt vets and their wives couldn't be regularly collecting piglets from the public highway, so a few weeks later, with some relief that was nevertheless tinged with regret, we bade farewell to our two sows as they departed for the market. Our pig-farming days were over.

But we had also at the kennels a motley collection of feathered and furred fauna. The former were hens, 200 of them of different breeds, which I kept in the deep-litter system in a large shed. Since a lad, I'd always known hens about the place, and they were a decided source of revenue with a nice tidy profit – if you forgot the hours spent daily in washing eggs. As well as giving me endless pleasure in sitting of an evening watching them, they gave us some extra cash with which to equip our home with what we regarded as luxuries, but what certainly in today's world would be considered necessities. After having electricity installed in the house, the poultry profit provided a brand-new electric cooker to replace the enormous gas monstrosity we had purchased at a saleroom for £5. I recall yet the pleasure the purchase of that new cooker gave us; it was virtually the first new article we'd bought for our home since we'd set up poultry, with their easily available food and warm, deep bed of moss litter, attracted still more. Of course we tried the Pest Control Officer, but with so many dogs around he could not use poison readily, and there were too many exits to use traps effectively. Clearly, if there was to be any action it had to come from us. Regularly of an evening, father, mother and the two under-fives, Neil and Ian, would sally forth to a rat hunt; our first two offspring, it seemed to me as the months passed, had some terrier blood in them somewhere. We would all don wellington boots, tuck trouser legs into stockings, and wear gloves. I was armed with a large garden fork or spade for digging purposes, while the rest of the army sported long sticks or shovels. There was a surprise diversion one evening when Mum, who kept her boots in a shed at the back door, eased her feet into them. She suddenly leapt skywards, and to the infinite amusement of our senior boy, Neil, aged four, gave a very passable demonstration of a Zulu war dance, complete with yells. It was only when she succeeded in kicking off her boots and one somewhat dazed rat staggered out that we learnt the reason for the antics. Mercifully she had not been bitten, but ugh! . . . even to step on one of the squirming brutes! Then we would proceed in formation to the deep-litter house, and while father dug out the obvious tunnels, mother and children would guard the escape routes. Those brown rats which escaped my weapon were enthusiastically chased by the family with loud yells, shouts and the thump of descending sticks, all to a deafening background of cackles, cries and fluttering from the poultry. Our record kill was thirty-nine in one night. We never completely mastered them, only kept them within bounds, but in the process we probably completely ruined our sons for life, what with yells of 'Shut up!' and 'There he's; hit him!'

But, of course, kennels are the dwelling places of dogs, and our inmates came into one of three groups:

'Yes, it's usual for a few days after surgery,' I replied, equally flummoxed.

'Has she been ill, then?' he inquired.

'We-ell, not ill. Just a bit quiet for a few days. That's usual after an op.'

'Operation for what?' he persisted.

It was becoming increasingly obvious to me that our lines had become crossed, and equally increasingly I feared what would be revealed when the tangle was unravelled.

'The operation you asked for, the spay, the sterilization,' I said guardedly.

He looked at me a long time, at least thirty minutes, I'm sure! Or so it felt before he snapped, 'I said no such thing!' I couldn't really blame him for snapping; I'd have bitten in the circumstances.

'Well, Mr Mooney, I'm very sorry indeed, but the message I received was that Paula was in for a spay and would be collected in ten days. If something is amiss, I can only apologize.'

'I said she was in for a *stay* – and would be collected in ten days.'

He was a well-to-do hotelier and could afford a dozen pedigree boxers, but that was beside the point. Paula was his pride and joy, he'd planned to let her have pups, and we'd ruined his plans. I must say he took it astonishingly well, for she was a really lovely animal. I suppose he might have sued us, but he didn't. It was a genuine telephone-message mistake, and he did have a rather quiet voice. Needless to say, there was no charge for either spay or stay! He even forgave us, and boarded Paula with us again. I suppose he reasoned that we couldn't do any more damage.

Many of the second group, the boarders, were regulars year after year, and sometimes several times a year. Some owners even reserved certain kennels, and the majority of their pets settled in reasonably well to communal life. Many almost on the point of collapse, but assured me a neighbour was driving her home; we sent her off, took the little fellow in, and within minutes had him out of his world of pain, if only for a time. Mrs Kerr had told us before departing that she had been away all morning and had come home to be told by a neighbour that an alsatian had attacked Chota. Then the little fellow had disappeared. It was evident from this account that the eye had been displaced at least five hours before, and the amount of swelling confirmed this. I vaguely recalled that the surgery book had indicated that, if treated in time, it was sometimes possible to replace the eyeball in its socket; we could but try.

As usual, Mrs Drury, our efficient assistant cum secretary, was unflappable, as if eyes lying about were an everyday occurrence. She watched the anaesthetic, and from the other side of the table was ready, as always, to give me whatever instrument I might require. That I didn't yet know. I had, of course, removed a few diseased or badly damaged eyes before, but I confess I quailed before that eye, staring fixedly at me from its resting place on the dog's cheek, as if daring me to touch it while its owner was out for the count. But touch it we did, gently bathing and cleaning. Then, with plenty of antiseptic cream for lubrication, lashings of patience, and firm but gentle pressure, I tried to coax the eyeball back.

'He's coming round,' said Mrs Dru's voice.

'We can't have that; more Pentothal, Mrs D.' She moved to get it.

My normal form of anaesthesia for reasonably short operations was Pentothal (the so-called 'truth drug'), followed by a mask with ether–oxygen mixture to keep the patient at the desired depth of unconsciousness. But to fix a face-mask to a snub-nosed dog was difficult – to one with an eyeball lying on its face, impossible. So more Pentothal was put in a vein. I cannot recall now how long we worked on boarding space. It was the height of summer, we were very full, but we made room. They were humble folk, and told us that they came from Wolverhampton, and that the dog was called Whisky. He proved to be a Grade A, Category 1 nuisance, a barker with a capital B. Fortunately for everyone's peace of mind, most days his owners took him off our hands to return him in the evenings, when he proceeded to bark incessantly at all and sundry, albeit wagging his tail as if to say, 'No offence, chums.' But it was apparent that Sandy had taken offence. I imagine he had told the new arrival to pipe down, and had been, from the safety of his strong, Sandy-proof kennel, told where to get off by Whisky. Nobody spoke to Sandy like that in any language; it was doubly insulting to his West Country nature to be addressed in the language of Wolverhampton! Sandy morosely brooded, and thought dark thoughts. During morning exercise one day, Sandy had a go at Whisky, who, not imbued with the spirit from which he took his name, fled for dear life. Fortunately the chase was spotted and Sandy restrained in time. But he waited, glaring and muttering threats at this upstart, who – brave as always in his secure kennel – barked back his abuse.

There came a day when Whisky's owners left him behind while they went on a coach trip. All was peaceful in the warmth of a Devon summer afternoon, thought Janet as she pottered in the little garden between rests in a deck-chair, for in a few days our next babe was due. Suddenly the summer calm was shattered by a growl, then a scream, followed by the barking of every dog in the kennels. Hurrying as fast as circumstances would allow, Janet went into the kennels. Somehow, Sandy had escaped from his pen, managed to get into Whisky's and had him pinned to the ground. The poor girl fled for the phone, to be told at the surgery that both vets were miles away in the country. She had it all to sort out herself. Hardly realizing what she was doing, she struck and

There was the young St Bernard who came to be boarded for a fortnight, his front legs resplendent in full-length leather boots, which his own vet had recommended for a tendency to rickets – for, as everyone knows, a St Bernard with rickets would not be much cop carrying his barrel up Mont Blanc to succour some stranded mountaineer. We had another St Bernard, Carlo, who boarded with us for a year, a great, lolloping hunk of good nature. His owners had moved to London and it was a full twelve months before they could find premises suitable to have him with them again. Then there was Boris the borzoi. Like Carlo, he was with us a very long time (I forget now why; something about an owner going overseas), but there the resemblance ended. Carlo was everybody's friend, Boris nobody's. Carlo was one of the gang; Boris would not so demean himself. He was evidently a pre-Revolution borzoi, a real czar, who went about on his own every day from first to last, with his nose in the air. None of your proletarians for Boris! He didn't even sleep beside them, apparently preferring the side of the kennels which was seldom used and where he could keep his own company. I did not like the dog, but I was sorry for him. He reminded me of some European monarch, displaced from his throne and with nowhere to go.

But of all our characters, Cindy was the favourite. She was a gentle brown, black and white mongrel, with hints of spaniel, sheepdog and foxhound blood in her, and maybe a dash of some kind of terrier far back. She came to us as a tiny puppy, one of eight that had been found, with their mother, under a hedge, and rescued by the RSPCA Inspector. The mother made a good job of rearing her large brood, and quite quickly she herself and seven of the puppies had found good homes. One little one was left: Cindy. She grew, appeared regularly in the papers with the others in the 'Good homes wanted' column, but nobody wanted Cindy. She was nobody's child. She saw other waifs come and go, replacement. His eyes wandered over a collie, a labrador, an alsatian, then stopped at Cindy. His face lit up. 'That's the one,' he said, and as if she knew it, Cindy stood on her hind legs to greet him. The stranger had at last come in from the cold.

The kennels were a bind, often a nuisance, sometimes a heartbreak, but when I saw Cindy go off into the new life with a real master, I thought of the joys we also knew with our dogs. Cindy never came back. She had no need to, not ever again.

ours, were not settled then – they were not settled till next Season.

I knew that the town and its adjacent caravan sites were filling up, but as I passed our waiting-room for afternoon consulting hour one spring day, I knew without question that the Season was upon us once more, for the room was full, and half the customers seemed to be poodles. The poodle was the in breed of the decade. We had quite a few as permanent residents in the town, but the poodle population multiplied enormously with the coming of summer. I wasn't too fond of the breed – a nice enough and quite intelligent wee dog, but some a bit neurotic, like half the owners! The only dog I'd seen go completely round the bend had been a poodle, after producing a litter of pups. The strain of motherhood seemed to unhinge completely what brain it possessed, and though in a human mother post-natal depression was fairly common, I'd never heard of post-natal hysteria until seeing it in that poodle. The wretched little creature howled incessantly, an unearthly kind of screech that caused the occupants of houses within a hundred yards of the locus to talk of mass evacuation, or poodle-icide! We'd had to keep the dog under morphia, no less, for a week, all other tranquillizers or sedatives proving powerless against that appalling cry.

Sure enough, the first case that day was a white poodle, carried by a glamorous blonde. Though it was a warm day, she was sheathed in a fur coat, her companion dressed in a pink ribbon. I recognized the glamour girl as Tanya or Melinda or some such name, the leading lady of the summer show in the Pavilion. She had been here last year, too. In a voice so refined that I could only comprehend about every fourth word, she gave me to understand that Chi-Chi's blood seemed overheated and she was scratching herself more or less non-stop.

I assured her our little secret was safe, and so it has been, until now.

I understood the reason for the tender appeal bit, for the next customer was also from the summer show, and also a poodle owner. She was, I imagined, one of the chorus girls, and came clad in just the bare minimum allowable for appearing in the street. I didn't know what her stage name was, but as soon as she opened her mouth I recognized her place of origin. I grinned and asked, 'What part of Glasgow are you from?'

'Hill Street,' she replied. I told her I had been to the college in Buccleugh Street, which was next to Hill Street. We said 'Fancy that' and 'It's a wee world', 'Just imagine' and 'Would you credit that', then the lady informed me, 'We used tae see the greyhounds goin' in there, so we did, but we never saw ony come oot.' She was right, too. The penalty for being an unsuccessful greyhound was to end up an anatomy specimen in Buccleugh Street!

'I've just had another member of your cast in,' I told her.

'Och, aye – Tanya!' (or it may have been Melinda). 'She's frae Glesca tae.'

'No!'

'Aye!'

'She doesn't sound like it.'

'Maybe no' in here; she can fair pit on the la-di-da, but you should hear her when she's no' pleased – pure Gallagate then! Her richt name's Annie McGonigle. Me, a'm Mary Bell, but a'm jist in the chorus so a don't need a fancy name. Whit wis wrang wi' her dug? She said it wis its high breedin', that the bluid wis ower rich – wis that richt?'

Mindful of my promise, and of professional etiquette, I hastily changed the subject. 'And what's wrong wi' your wee dog?'

Sexing mice, let alone newly-born ones, was an original request.

The wee hand was clutching a minute purse. 'How many pennieth ith that?' she inquired.

I grinned at her, and handed back the box. 'You keep your pennieth . . . eh . . . your money; that's all right, my dear.'

The next customer was a boy with a tortoise.

'It's got a sore eye,' he announced.

I peered at the beast. I was willing to believe him, but at the moment its head was inside the shell, and no eye visible. I poked at it and nothing happened. I knocked on the shell; it did not answer my knock. I hadn't at that time treated many tortoises, in fact the last one had been brought, not for treatment, but to be put to sleep. Its owner had rung up in horror to say that her tortoise had just come out of hibernation minus three legs, which had been eaten by a rat, and what was she to do. My wife had advised her to hit it on the head! Apart from the difficulty of such a feat, I'd had to administer a gentle rebuke that you didn't speak to clients that way. The poor creature had been brought in, and we'd chloroformed it and put it out of its misery. I remember initially trying to get its head out – though I hadn't tried hitting it on the skull.

'Look, son,' I said in my most professional manner, 'I think it will be best if you go back to the waiting-room, and my assistant will help me to do this.'

So, summoning Mrs Drury from her desk, I turned to her in the surgery and asked, 'Any ideas on how to make a tortoise stick its head out? What does Major Davidson do?'

For once, that mine of information was stumped. It seemed that Kenneth's and Mrs Drury's lives had been pretty well tortoise-free too, and so far as veterinary husbandry, surgical and medical textbooks were concerned, the tortoise had apparently not been invented when they were fact, witnessing this sickening spectacle several times, I had felt that someone ought to put in a public plea for male lib.

'Would you care to show me the lump?' I asked the lady, for nothing was very obvious through the hair.

'Charles, show the veterinary doctor the lump.'

At the command, Charles leapt into action, scrabbled about among the hair, and pointed. I wondered if Charles was naturally dumb, or only when his wife was present to speak for both of them.

'When did you notice this?' I asked.

'Only this morning. It was horrible then, and has grown since,' said the Speaker.

'And it will go on growing too!' I said.

'Oh, dearie me,' she wailed in a high soprano – surprising really, for with her build I'd have thought she was more a contralto, if not actually a baritone. She wrung her hands, and I gazed fascinated, for this action was often referred to in melodramas, but seldom actually seen. It produced quite a clink and jingle as her many bangles, rings and trinkets met head on. 'Can nothing be done?' she bayed.

'Oh, yes, quite easily. I expect you were walking on the Torrs yesterday?'

'Oh, you wonderful man! How did you guess?' She gazed at me in wonderment, and for one awful moment I thought she was about to embrace me, so I backed away hurriedly and picked up a pair of forceps. I dare say it was all right for her to embrace Charles, if she ever did, for he only came up to her shoulder, but since I was as tall as Charles's owner, I feared for my ribs in such a bear hug.

'Now, don't worry if your dog gives a little yelp. I'm about to pull the lump out' – and before she could protest at this cruel act, I did it, and held it up for her to see.

'It's a tick . . . very common around here, especially on the Torrs. They fasten on to sheep, dogs, or any animal, and suck its blood, and so grow quite dramatically – something

That seemed to be the lot, and I was just taking off my white coat, preparatory to starting the afternoon visits, when the door burst open and the blue poodle owner and little Charles bearing the dog arrived again in a state of near hysteria. Dinkums, it appeared, had suddenly gone round the bend. They'd returned to their nearby boarding house, and the lady had proceeded forthwith to reward her brave little dog with a slap-up feed, when poppet, or baa-lamb, or whoever he was, had quite suddenly rushed round the room, yelping, pawing his mouth, rolling over, jumping up, and generally giving every sign of having flipped his lid. The battle cruiser seemed about to do likewise, or explode any minute, so I called to Mrs Drury to take her into the waiting-room and calm her.

'Sit on her, if you need to, but keep her out of the surgery,' I whispered. Mrs Drury, who was about a third the size of Charles's helpmeet, gave me a pained look which I took to mean that the odds were hardly fair – a bantamweight taking on a heavy. 'You can cope,' I assured her with a smile, as she led the sobbing lady by the arm, like a tug with a liner in tow.

'Now, Mr . . . er . . . Charles; let's have a look at your dog!'

I prised open the poppet's mouth, then reached for the forceps again, stronger ones this time. I'd guessed what I would find, the description being fairly typical of the trouble.

'Hold him tightly,' I said.

The little man did this with great gusto, gripping the dog by the scruff of the neck in a manner I'm sure his lady would not have liked at all, and which caused the dog to yelp loudly. Charles seemed to be enjoying it too. I only hoped Mrs Drury was sitting firmly on the lady next door. I fancy if she'd appeared and seen her man getting down to things, and doing what he'd clearly wanted to do for some time to

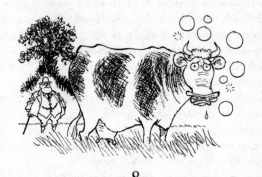

8

The Volks from Away

'Hello! Is thack the veterererinary . . . (click) . . . surgeon?'

'Yes – Cameron here.' I was trying to place the voice, with its odd clipped pronunciation and background of clicks.

'This is Mr Badger.' Ah, I had it now. Mr Badger had considerable trouble with his dentures, which at times stuck out like a boxer's gum-shield, and when he made a speech of any length they slid up and down, clicking like castanets. He must have had these teeth for forty years.

'What can I do for you, Mr Badger?'

'I do nock know if you can do anythink.'

'As bad as that, eh? Well, what does the trouble seem to be?'

'I very much fear I have foot . . . (click) . . . and mouth disease.'

'You have foot and mouth, do you say?' I knew about the mouth . . . the foot was a new development.

Edwin Badger. He was one of the large contingent in the area who were described by the Devonians as 'the volks from away'. 'Away' was a delightfully vague term denoting Somerset, Scotland or Swaziland. If you weren't from North Devon, you were from 'away'. This band of immigrants was a mixed bag. Some were officers from one of the three Services who had sunk their demob payment in a farm, and who for the most part were doing well; they were keen, intelligent, genned-up on their new life and willing to learn. We had farmers who had come from other parts of the country, and almost without exception they had proved outstanding. Although Devon was exceedingly beautiful and its land fertile, some of the farming methods were fairly primitive, and with the modern methods of the incomers allied to Devon's rich soil they very soon forged ahead. But there were others of humbler lineage from 'away'. By and large, these were 'volks' who had longed for a little place in the country, and in the glories of sunny Devon, with its gentle people and slower pace of life, they were enjoying a more leisurely, if at times uncertain, existence.

Mr Badger was of this latter breed. He was a retired greengrocer from London, who had apparently cherished a secret desire to settle down in the country and own his personal little piece of 'England's green and pleasant land'. With great daring he had taken the plunge, retired early and bought about fifteen acres. His smallholding was at Martincombe, that district of patchwork fields stretching up the steep surrounding hills, famed for its warm climate and early strawberries, and with a honeycomb of lanes leading to the various cottages and little farms which perched so precariously on ledges and outcrops that one felt that any sleepwalker stepping out of his front door would disappear into the abyss, and be gathered up, in whole or in part, hundreds of feet below.

I had only been at the Badger residence once before, and it

my spreading-joy-around tone, 'Nothing to worry about. No ulceration in foot or mouth. She has wooden tongue, due to a germ called *Actinobacillus lignieresi*, affecting the tongue and soft tissues around. I'll give her an injection, and leave you a bottle to give her a dose every day. In ten days or so, she'll be as sound as a bell.'

'But her sympcoms are so like foo . . . (click) . . . and mouth disease,' he said despondently. I think he was genuinely disappointed and had been looking forward to writing to some greengrocer friend, saying: 'Dear Jack (or Bill, or Bert), I'm afraid I've got bad news to report . . .'

'Well, Mr Badger, a lot of diseases have similar symptoms. If you look at a medical dictionary, you can imagine you have any number of things wrong with you, and rush off to make your Will.'

Over the ritual hand-washing in the kitchen, I inquired, 'How was the lambing this year?'

'Quite good,' he replied lugubriously (it would have been an education to find him on a bad day, I thought). 'We had ten twins, but the trouble is the ewes will keep lambing at night. However,' he added, some excitement coming into his voice and transforming his expression from deep solemnity to a kind of sombre deadpan look, 'I'm having no more lambings at night. Next year they will all lamb through the day.'

'Good for you!' I congratulated him. 'What's the secret?'

He looked at me rather pityingly, as if I should have known by now. 'Why, I'll only put the ram out with the ewes through the day this autumn, then all the lambs are bound to arrive by day. It's so simple, really!'

I tittered, then hastily changed it to a fit of coughing, for he was absolutely serious. Hastily, before I exploded, I bade them goodbye, then laughed non-stop for about three miles of my journey. A childless couple, they fondly imagined they had discovered a secret that had remained hidden from

'We've got the very pill for you.' We had, in fact, an excellent diuretic which flushed out the kidneys like a hose! We had used it successfully on numerous dogs, and had even had success with stones in the kidneys, the drug appearing sometimes to dissolve or break up the calculi.

'Give me some to try,' he pleaded, and – foolishly – I did. I warned him that if anything went wrong he must contact his doctor and stop the pills right away, and left him. I'd been a worried man since, and had even scanned the obituary notices, fearful of finding his name. But he was still there, looking as grey as before, walking straddle-legged, and doubled up over the cow I'd come to see. I was sorry to find him like that, but relieved to find him there at all. Casually I asked, 'How did you get on with the pills?'

'Tremendous,' he said, 'they worked marvellously. The only trouble was that they brought such lumps of stone down, it took me about an hour to pass each one. I tell you, you could have put them in a rockery. Look!' – he rummaged in a waistcoat pocket – 'did you ever see anything like these?'

I goggled, and gulped 'Never!', then added hastily, 'I think you'd better stop these pills, and get to your doctor and ask for an X-ray.'

'Ach, doctors!' he snorted, condemning the whole medical profession in two words. I talked to him for a time, managed to persuade him to do as I suggested, relieved him of the remainder of my pills, and went on my way, considerably shaken by the jagged calculi the old man had passed.

As it happened, my next call was actually to a doctor's farm. Dr White was an easy-going, friendly soul, with a limitless fund of stories. He had retired relatively young from a busy Midlands practice and, with his Irish wife, kept about the muckiest farm in the area. It was quite a feat to walk across their yard without having a wellington sucked off in the slime! I was constantly surprised at the cases to that what with Badger's cure for night lambings, and the Pole's insistence that if a doctor said a day he should keep to it, sex education had been badly neglected in our land. I was spared any further 'Revelations of a Midlands Doctor' by Mrs White coming with a message that I was to go with all speed to Major Biggleswade's farm, where four heifers had been found dead and some others were very bad. Hastily washing my arms, I leapt into my jacket and my car, and put my foot down. Four dead — what could it be? Staggers, possibly . . . bloat, unlikely . . . what? The yearlings had apparently died without a struggle, as if poleaxed. A further half-dozen were staggering about, or were down, twitching and groaning.

There was a fair old hiatus, those awful few moments when the vet is surrounded by a sea of anxious faces, waiting for some word of hope. Major Biggleswade, another of our 'from away' people, was a first-class farmer, who had but recently moved from a small farm to a large one, indeed one of the best in the district. He tended to get a bit red in the face when agitated, and he had every reason to be bright red now. Four fine, fat, Devon yearlings was a considerable loss — another six would be catastrophic. At such a time the old grey matter is strained to the limit, as one attempts to recall, and mentally tick off, all the differential diagnostic features. Botulism . . . anthrax . . . magnesium deficiency . . . lightning stroke or electrocution . . . There was just nothing to be seen externally. It could only be a poison of some sort, I thought, and my heart, already pretty low, went right down into my boots, for the world of poisons — apart from reasonably obvious ones like bracken or lead — was a maze. The toxicology book was a most discouraging thing to read because most of the poisons had similar symptoms, most resulted in death, and in the vast majority of instances the book mournfully recorded that treatment was unavailing and a positive diagnosis could only be made

We injected the six survivors with adrenaline, then poured all the purgatives I had in my car over the poor beasts' throats – linseed oil, epsom salts, a bloat mixture with turpentine in it: everything remotely resembling a purge, proven and unproven, went over to try to shift that yew quickly, but I feared it was a hopeless business. I stayed a while, then went home, ostensibly for a meal but in reality to look up the poisons book. It was cheerful! It seemed that yew was invariably fatal, but a case had been recorded in 1859 when somebody had saved a beast. As an added item of interest, the author further informed us that yew poisoning also occurred in man, but only in lunatics! I've often ridiculed the reports in newspapers that 'doctors were fighting to save' somebody or other. Whenever somebody is ill, it appears that doctors don't simply treat, they battle for the patient's life. We did actually fight for these beasts' lives, almost hourly keeping them going with stimulants, in the hope that our various charges of dynamite would work in time. Two more died, four survived . . . just . . . and had diarrhoea for about a fortnight. But they lived.

So, in the ever-changing kaleidoscope that made up our lives, I had spent an afternoon with 'the volks from away'. I had begun with a serious disease that wasn't; I had learnt the great secret of day-time lambings; I had learnt how not to treat humans for renal calculi, and how not to predict a delivery date; and I had learnt how to face crisis and loss with dignity, as Major Biggleswade had done.

The men of Devon were, and are, a delightful, friendly race. Their rich, rolling tongue is music in the ear. But in the main, critical as it may seem, the farming standards in Devon thirty years ago were poor and primitive, and their improvement is certainly due, in part, to 'the volks from away'. Of that I'm 'sartin sure, m'dears'!

College, and while I had remained doucely in my native
Ayrshire as an assistant, Jimmy had departed for the warmer
clime of Somerset, there to learn the trade – and, I've no
doubt, cause a flutter in a few feminine hearts, for there's no
doubt he was a real charmer, was Jimmy. We didn't corre-
spond very often, but out of the blue came this racy letter
from him, most of which, in the manner of assistants in
every profession from time immemorial, had been devoted
to slanging his boss in carefully chosen, selective but
definitely vitriolic terms, reaching his most outright condemnation with the reference to crowbars. No, I couldn't
imagine quite, at that stage of my experience, how crowbars
could ever be necessary in calving a poor beast, but there and
then, as Jimmy had already clearly decided, I vowed with all
the confidence of the inexperienced that there would never
be a time when I would need to use such force. Never!
Never! On that I was quite clear.

But times change, and the stage of seeing everything as
black or white tends to pass in the arena of bitter experience.
The passing years have a habit of making us swallow our
words as we realize how much we still don't know, and
Jimmy's reference to crowbars came vividly back to me
some years later.

I was in bed, tucked up with hot-water bottles, having
alternated the previous day between penicillin pills, throat
lozenges and a cough bottle. I had flu, and none of your
forty-eight-hour varieties either! In fact as I lay sweating it
out, it came to me that maybe I should have made my Will,
but since my life insurance was already being used as cover
for the cost of my partnership in the practice of Davidson
and Cameron, there didn't seem much point in a Will. I
would either have to get better, or (as seemed more likely)
quietly decease, and hope there would be enough somewhere for the funeral. While in this cheerful frame of mind,
the phone rang.

The fine modern cowshed was warm after the night air, warm and aromatic with that lovely mixture of smells that pervades a byre – hay, silage, cattle cake, the animals themselves – a smell that always made it feel good to be a vet, working with living things. But not that night; the magic failed to work its spell, for I couldn't get over my own wretchedness and the shivers were coming continuously as I struggled into my calving-coat. Soaping the arm – at least the bucket of water was warm – I examined the patient. Farmer Parkhurst was quite right: the calf was coming normally. It was also large, very large, and big, roomy and strong as the Friesian was, she was not going to deliver this calf unaided. I got the calving-chains on and tried a bit of traction. I had about as much strength as a newborn kitten!

'Can you give a bit of a pull here?'

'I can't,' said Mr Parkhurst, 'I'm only a week out of hospital after a hernia. But Andrew can lend a hand.' I said I was sorry about his operation, groaned inwardly and looked at Andrew, all in the one go. Andrew was a big lad, the oldest of the Parkhurst boys, but he was only fifteen. Andrew and I pulled on the chains, the cow bellowed and strained, but the calf came not an inch.

'All we need is a strong pull here. Can you get any helpers?' I asked.

'Not at this time of night,' he replied, shaking his head.

'Then we're in trouble,' I said. 'This calf is going to take some shifting; you daren't pull, I've got the flu and that leaves one fit man, Andrew.'

(Here let me insert an explanation. I have often noticed a look of horror come over the face of the layman when I describe a calving. I have seen the word 'barbaric' form in the mind, as they think of maybe six men pulling on ropes or calving-chains to deliver a calf. In defence of the veterinary profession vis-à-vis the medical, I would explain that the vet cannot, as with a human mother, arrange a half-ton cow in

'Now then, Andrew,' I explained to the son, 'you're the important one here tonight. Do exactly as I say. When I say "stop", you stop at once. When I say "steady", I mean an inch at a time. Can you handle it?'

There was a flicker of eagerness on the boy's face, but he immediately got rid of it. I thought as I looked from father to son that I had seldom seen such a pair of dour Devonians. I don't know why, but they reminded me of Scrooge, the bad Scrooge at the beginning of Dickens's *Christmas Carol*, only they were more full and fair of face than the old miser. I suppose my subconscious was recalling to me the reluctance of all the Parkhursts to pay their bills – or maybe I was delirious! Stop dreaming, I chided myself, and get on with it.

'Well then, lad, let's have it,' I said.

Soon a roar was heard as the tractor was started, the byre door flung open to admit a blast of freezing air and choking diesel fumes as the boy reversed his mechanical steed right up to the door, and through it. The door was wide, the cow was right opposite it, which saved a bit of shifting around, and operation Broken Vow was about to commence. The leg calving-chains were fixed together to the tractor towbar, and when I repeated, 'An inch at a time, mind you,' young Andrew nodded and did just that, while I, with my hand inside the cow, felt for progress and tried to guide the direction of pull. I felt the legs budge and move up into position, yelled 'Stop!', and at once the tractor stopped.

'Now for the tricky bit, the head,' I shouted over the tractor's roar. As with the legs, now the head chain alone was linked to the drawbar, and I nodded. I glanced at Mr Parkhurst and thought he'd be back in hospital shortly at this rate, for his chin was almost tripping him. To say he didn't like it was fractionally an understatement! But Andrew was inching forward, and I soon had other things on my mind than Parkhurst's long face, as I tried to guide a very broad face into the mouth of the uterus and up into the

Andrew! Great driving, lad!' at which the boy, forgetting for a moment the code of the Parkhursts, actually smiled.

As I made my weary way homeward, I reflected on the events just past. I shuddered to think what might have happened if the driver's foot had slipped on the clutch, but otherwise I was not too morose at having broken one of my self-imposed commands. A 'never' had gone for a burton, but in retrospect it seemed to me that a steady, controlled pull had been much more effective, and quicker, than six pairs of hands tugging at ropes. Jimmy's boss had known what he was about when he used a crowbar, calving-ropes attached, as a lever, no doubt against the concrete lip of the dung channel.

Flu or not, I was out early next day, fearful lest something had overtaken my patient. I needn't have worried. She was lying down, chewing the cud, having evidently had a hearty breakfast, which was more than I'd had. Parkhurst senior was with me, and as he looked at the beast and at me, he observed, 'She's looking better than you are, Mr Cameron!' I thought wryly that wouldn't be hard. Clearly we need worry no more about the patient. In fact, my only concern now was what farmer Parkhurst would deduct from the calving fee for diesel and use of tractor!

The trouble with one 'never' going down the drain is that others are sure to follow. It's a bit like an alcoholic; the first drink is one too many and opens the floodgates. Accompanied by two students, one a coloured lad from Nigeria and the other a Scot, I was right out at the fringe of the practice on the moor. Here several veterinary practices met, all roughly the same distance from home, so in each case the various farmers would compare notes as to how their own vet did the job. One of my moorland clients was Hockridge, and a rougher establishment would be hard to imagine. It textbooks on hygiene and animal husbandry – of up-to-date crushes, gathering and shedding pens, a concrete yard which could be hosed afterwards, and a little niche for the vet beside the crush where, in safety and some degree of comfort, he could do his job. Instead, before them stretched a sea of sweating bovine backs, their owners kicking and plunging about, while outside the stockade a group of men with sticks and curses sought to prevent the beasts leaning on their home-made restraining wall. Since the two lads were going to assist me with finding the ear marks and noting down the identification individually, they realized that they had to enter the arena. Over the wall we went, and I heard one of them mutter, 'Now I know what the Christians felt like, facing the Roman lions.' Still in one piece, but having accumulated a few kicks and much dirt on our various persons, we reached our point of operations.

'Let's try and do the Galloways first while they are still packed in,' I bellowed at Hockridge, who nodded. But between the concept of any great plan and its fulfilment, there is many a snag. So it was to prove. The only way to get a beast into the crush was for one of the men in the bunch to take its tail, and with the assistance of others, manhandle it to where we awaited it. The more manhandling that went on inside, the more the beasts pressed on the restraining five-bar gates, the result being that those helpers outside cursed those inside, while these sweating, dung-covered figures cursed back. Since most of the words were in broad Devonian – and some of them new to me – and with the snorts and roars all around, fortunately all was not understood by my two lads, the Nigerian merely observing, 'I think they are swearing quite a lot!' He sure hit the target; in fact if all that was said and shouted that afternoon was written down, this chronicle would be ten times as long.

125

'Reckon about two days, since she started, like.'

Lying in front of us, on a bed of filth, was a heifer having her first calf. She was lying on her side, but stretched full out, so that her chain (incongruously the one secure beast was chained) was all but throttling her. The heifer was far through, and protruding from her were the head and fore-limbs of her calf. Two days, I thought – by the smell, more like two weeks. This was a typical piece of Hock-ridge neglect. I whirled round on him, demanding, 'Why did you not call us before?' to which he replied, again typically, 'Reckoned since you was comin' anyways, might as well wait and get the visit paid by the government, like.'

I thought of the lecturer who had told us that we would probably have to educate some of our clients. I wonder where he would have begun with Hockridge.

'Look,' I said, 'there's one of three things we can do here. One: shoot the cow. Two: do an embryotomy and cut the calf up into bits. Three: try to calve it. I'd suggest to shoot her would be a kindness.'

'Nor, she be out of a good 'un an' I'd like to save her,' he answered. Clearly this was to be his milk cow, since every other hoofed creature was out on the moor.

'Right then!' I glared at him. 'Plenty of hot water, soap, towel, and quickly.'

'Ain't no hot water in house.'

'Then boil some – plenty.'

We waited, already tired, dirty, dishevelled. There was no offer of tea – we were out in the wilds. I looked at the two students, both silent, both experiencing for the first time how crude their future calling could sometimes be.

'You know,' I said with an attempt at cheerfulness, 'the first vet I saw practice with used to say: "You may not see much practice, but you will see life." You've been in my lady's chamber, to treat her darling little King Charles students had gone by then, though sorry they did not see Hockridge's heifer – for she recovered, astonishingly, and he paid a whopping bill! That was the only way I knew to educate this client.

My last 'never' to disappear left me with a red face. Jim Glover, whose shop was just across from our surgery, breezed in one teatime and said, 'Alex. Could you spare a minute to look at my old bitch? There's something not right about her.'

I nipped over the way and saw Jim's whippet, which was wandering about aimlessly, her back slightly arched. I took her temperature and noticed there was a slight uterine discharge. Then I palpated her abdomen, and asked Jim if she'd ever had pups. Her abdomen was certainly enlarged a bit.

'No.'

'When was she last in season?'

'I can't remember; ages ago. She's so old I think she's stopped.'

'Well, Jim,' I said quite confidently, 'she's got a condition called pyometra, very common in maiden bitches. Her womb is swollen, but not too big, and some discharge is coming away. It might mean a hysterectomy, but we'll try some tablets first, at her age.'

'Right, Alex,' said Jim, and came over for the tablets.

The next morning at nine a.m., Jim walked in again in his usual jovial manner and reported.

'Alex. I thought you'd like to know that the whippet had a pup through the night. Will she still need that operation, do you think?'

'Er, no, Jim . . . I think the womb will be OK now.'

I heard an echo over the years from the old Vet College: 'When you are asked by an examiner for the causes of enlargement of the abdomen in a bitch, along with enlarged

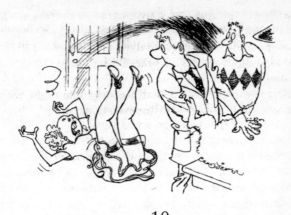

10

Surprises of a Caesar

I came out of the shop, turned left, and started to make my way back to the surgery. I'd been to the barber's shop for a much-needed haircut, for what with lambings, calvings, tuberculin tests and all the rush of the spring work, I'd had little time for any 'short back and sides'. However, a glance in the mirror that morning had startled me to the point of realizing that if I didn't have it done soon, I'd either need to go round the various hairdressers and ask for an estimate, or let somebody have a go with sheep shears. I had an operation scheduled for four o'clock, but until then I was free. So after our post-lunch conference and time of fellowship, I left Bernard, my new partner, to cope with afternoon consulting time and any subsequent calls, and wandered along to my hairdresser.

Barbers' shops are great places for brushing up on the local news, so it was with my knowledge much increased and thatch much diminished that I started back along the matter of cause and effect. The initial cause in this instance was that outside our door was parked Bernard's car, a perfectly proper and safe place to leave it. However, in front of Bernard's Ford was a client's Land-Rover, while in front of that again was a car and trailer with my four o'clock patient arriving. Opposite the three cars was parked a butcher's van, thus considerably narrowing the space through which other vehicles could proceed, but all would have been well had not a large touring coach tried to negotiate the gap, thought better of it, and just sat there, waiting for something to happen. Around this convoy of vehicles quite a little crowd had gathered, including many of the bus tourists, watching a farmer emerge from our front door propelling a sheep, followed by Bernard with a snowy white lamb tucked under each arm. The situation was further confused by my four o'clock farmer trying to direct *his* sheep in through the door, while the onlookers watched with great interest, even clicking their cameras, convinced that this was one of the tourist attractions of Devon.

Now, had it not been that the Easter weekend was early this year, there would not have been so many cars and coaches about, getting themselves intermingled with our lambing season. This could be regarded as one cause, yet from another viewpoint, had not my client arrived with his sheep at the very moment another was departing with sheep and lambs, there would have been nothing to see, the coach would probably have managed to squeeze through, and there would have been no crowd of spectators. Or yet again, if the client of the first part – he whose lambs Bernard was depositing in the Land-Rover beside their bleating mother – had phoned to make an appointment, this clash of comings and goings could have been averted, but being one of the easy-going Tuckers he had just – typically – arrived unannounced. Or – pursuing our quest for the cause of chaos even further – had we not, as a partnership, acquired the vagina, a common occurrence which rendered normal lambing difficult, if not brutal.

Principally, though, we did caesars in such volume because of a condition known as ringwomb, and surprise of surprises, there wasn't any such condition, said the pundits. When Kenneth had first written to the *Veterinary Record* of the condition he had been answered in strong terms by one of the best-known vets in the country, who firmly declared that after many years in practice he had never come across 'this so-called ringwomb', and suggested that if the sheep were left alone, they would lamb normally. He said, in effect, that Kenneth was rushing his fences, and his 'ringwomb' was merely a stage maybe twenty-four hours before full term and a normal birth. Letters flowed in week after week taking sides in the debate and suggesting all manner of remedies, most of which we'd tried without success. What we described as ringwomb was a condition where a ewe came into labour normally, at full term, but where the os (the mouth of the uterus) simply did not open, or open enough, to allow steerage way for the oncoming lamb. Examination of these ewes revealed a hard ring, the os, either completely closed or only slightly open, and no matter how long we'd left the ewe, the condition had persisted. I'd seen ewes in labour for days, and die with the womb still closed, the 'ring' remaining firm. We'd thought it was a hormone deficiency, but none of the oestrogens or sex hormones had proved successful. Someone had reported success with spinal anaesthesia – the idea being, I suppose, that this removed pain and allowed relaxation of the muscles – but it hadn't worked for us. Since Hoare's *Veterinary Therapeutics* informed us that 'in functional constriction of the cervix uteri, extract of belladonna freely applied might overcome the spasm and allow delivery to take place', we'd tried belladonna, with little result. In fact, short of 'eye of newt, skin of frog, web of spider and cow parsley there was a risk of total loss, well, there would be that anyway if she was left alone, slaughter in that state bringing at most £2. Clearly, reasoned the farming community, there was money in it, and the news caused a stirring of interest akin to a miniature gold rush in men who would never previously have dreamed of taking a mere sheep to a vet.

The second factor was that Major Kenneth Davidson was a superb surgeon, his big, beefy hands being remarkably swift and dexterous, in full control of his task. Compared with him I was at first a ham-fisted bungler, but I learnt much from watching and assisting him at work. Perhaps I never matched him, for he was a born surgeon while I was a vet who did surgery out of necessity, preferring diagnosis and medical treatment to knife work; yet in time apparently it was said that 'the Scottish vet'nary be all right, nigh as good's Major'. Bernard, however, having seen much practice with us as a student and then succeeding Kenneth in the practice, was accepted from the beginning as having been well trained.

At first everything was carried out on the farm, sometimes on the kitchen table, more often on bales of straw in a draughty barn by the light of a Tilly lamp, or in an even more exposed corner of a hayshed where the lambing pens were sited so that one worked with an audience enthusiastically bleating either in praise or criticism. In those early days, too, the operation was carried out under a general anaesthetic, using chloral hydrate intravenously. While results were encouraging, losses were heavier than we wanted, because with dirt or spiders' webs festooning the walls of the shed and straw getting into the wound, a wide selection of bugs abounded to cause sepsis. Also, with a drug like chloral hydrate the lambs were born anaesthetized, and if weakly (and usually they were in the early days before farmers were educated to send for us in time) they didn't come out of the

Street, thought he might relax briefly and view the proceedings. We also had a student seeing practice with us, as we invariably had in the spring. To complete the party, Jim Glover, our ebullient butcher from across the road, was there. Jim had quite a history. He had been a real Casanova and a plausible rogue until recently, when just sitting in church he had been converted – 'gone religious', they said – and it showed, to the extent that he now stayed with his own wife instead of somebody else's, came home sober and paid his debts, all to the great astonishment of his former associates. Jim had taken to coming in regularly for a chat, so his presence that afternoon meant we had quite an audience for theatre.

Now, at this point in the proceedings I think I should warn, as television announcers do from time to time, that 'in what follows there may be certain scenes that could upset some viewers', so if you are one of the faint-hearted you might be as well to skip a couple of pages!

The ewe having been ushered into the Operations Room in the midst of all this concourse, and the spectators having positioned themselves around, I took what was the first step, soaped my arm and examined her *per vaginam* to ascertain if she did in fact require surgery, or if the lamb could be delivered in normal fashion. This examination is not painful, but uncomfortable; just as the patient tenses himself, grips the arms of the chair tightly and fears the worst when the dentist says 'Open wide', and produces a strangled groan when the offending molar is tapped, so the ewe gave a slight grunt – when there was an almighty clatter, and I looked round to see the would-be nurse out cold. I hadn't done a thing; no knife had gleamed in the overhanging arc lamp; no blood had dripped to the ground, so I thought the girl's reaction boded ill for her nursing career. (In fact she did in time become an excellent nurse.) Mrs Drury, with perhaps just the suggestion of a flush colouring her cheeks, whether into the established routine, Mrs Drury on one side of the patient, myself on the other.

It's always difficult for a narrator to decide how much detail should be put into his narrative, but just in case any reader finds himself on some lonely island with a pregnant ewe requiring assistance, it might be as well to sketch in the main steps! First, the soft wool of the sheep's underbelly is plucked, then the remainder is soaped and shaved, and swabbed with antiseptic. Using a very short, fine needle, the skin is anaesthetized, then the muscles beneath, and finally, with a longer needle, right down to the peritoneum. All the sheep should feel is the first prick, and that was so in this case. Next, the operation cloths were clipped in position, leaving only the area for incision visible. I was conscious of six pairs of eyes watching closely.

Preliminaries over, we were ready to commence. Mrs Drury clapped a scalpel into my hand from our tray of sterilized instruments, and with one bold stroke the skin was incised. The sheep didn't feel a thing, but judging from the indrawn breaths I heard, others did – particularly when blood welled up, to be immediately swabbed by my assistant, allowing a clear view of the little bleeding vessels, which were clamped, but not before we lost one of our spectators. With a muttered 'Alex, I couldn't do that for a pension,' our butcher was off. Evidently Jim didn't go in for black puddings, or a wee drop of blood wouldn't have worried him! I next cut the muscles, then, carefully, the shining sheet of the peritoneum, looking for all the world like fine plastic. A loop of bowel popped up into the wound, which it had no right to do, and it was speedily put in its place. There beneath was the uterus, and gently one horn of its V-shape was brought through the incision to the exterior. A healthy uterus with a living lamb in it was always, to me, a thing of beauty, and normally I thrilled at this moment, seeing there the wonderfully soft yet strong organ the Creator had designed, with its

141

she would not leave the room – I'd be more likely to yield first!

'Not very nice, Mrs Dru, is it? It'll be touch and go with this one.'

'One of the worst we've had,' was all she said, snipping away at catgut as I completed the second row of inversion sutures in the uterus and tucked it back inside the abdomen. The rest was routine – nylon continuous sutures for peritoneum, then muscles, and finally my favourite mattress stitch for the skin. Then the whole area was thoroughly cleansed, and dusted with sulphonamide. Without my asking, she handed the loaded syringe of penicillin (the farmer would give the ewe an injection each day for a week), and asked, 'Phenergan?'

'Yes, the first danger here will be shock.' She knew my drill and drugs of choice. 'Some pituitrin, too, I think. It's a risk, but the sooner she's pushing out that muck, the better. I only hope the sutures hold.'

So it was done, the sheep lifted down – a very exhausted, ill sheep – and as I removed my gown and started scrubbing away the smell of death from my hands, my assistant was already at work disinfecting the table, gathering and cleaning instruments, and putting them into the sterilizer with fresh operation cloths and swabs. You never knew when they would be needed again. Feeling a bit fresher, I sallied forth to find the departed spectators and saw a horrible sight. The two Hawkins sons were sitting on the stairs leading to the upstairs flat, and they were green! It wasn't clear whether they were at the stage of sickness where they feared they would die, or at the next stage where they feared they would not die. Father was leaning against the outer door, and, though pale, he at least looked human. Our student was OK and making animated conversation with Mrs Drury's sister, who still seemed happy to lie on the couch. She got short shrift from her older sister. 'You still minutes and we had another little ewe with a very large lamb, a caesar having been performed in this case because the lamb's horns were so far developed that they were preventing passage through the vagina, a quite common occurrence in the Exmoor Horn hogg. These two had been a sheer delight to perform and one felt a sense of achievement, seeing two happy mothers, three healthy lambs and one satisfied farmer depart into the night; it provided a needed corrective after the seventy-minutes' struggle with death of the afternoon.

Well, the day was over, and as we gathered up instruments together I could steal a kiss from my present assistant, something that could not be done with the other, for either she or Janet, and probably both, would have up and dotted me one. Yes, there was something to be said for a husband and wife partnership, not to mention some early training for the family.

On the stroke of ten, we entered our living-room, just as the phone was ringing. It was Alf Spicer.

'Mr Cameron, uz's got a sheep right bad to lamb. Uz hears tell as how you'm got an operation that can save the lamb; be that right?'

'That's right, Alf, bring it in.'

Normally I didn't do caesars after ten o'clock, reasoning that they could wait till morning, but it was just ten now, our student was back, and I had him volunteer to come and assist. Out for tea, indeed, when other folk were working – where was the dedication in young vets nowadays! So the children were deposited in their beds once more, and after a cup of tea, Ian the student and I set out for positively the last caesar of the day, leaving instructions with Janet that if anyone called, there was Black Death in the town, or the 'vet'nary' had suspected rabies – anything to stall till morning. We delivered Alf's Border Leicester ewe of triplets, to his immense delight. I think he thought the operation was

There was no response. Bernard had a dazed look about him.

'Bernard!' I thundered, 'would you mind getting down here and work on saving these pups?'

'Eh?'

'These pups, Bernard, artificial respiration!'

'Oh, er, rather, I'm sure that's the right thing to do.'

'Then do it. Give Ann a hand with her pup.'

He was on his knees in a flash, his face wreathed in smiles as he knelt beside her.

After a time, I said, 'I think I can safely leave you two to cope now.'

'Rather!' said Bernard. 'I mean, we'll manage.'

And so they have, as man and wife, for many years. Yes, a caesar can produce many surprises, like target practice for Cupid, whose arrow, fired over a Yorkshire terrier and its puppies, unerringly found its mark that golden day.

might be all right for an olde-worlde, summertime-only residence, as a permanent home it left a lot to be desired. I had been to it once before when the former owner lived there, and I remember thinking initially it was the place the writer of the song 'Let the rest of the world go by' must have had in mind. It was, as the song described, 'a sweet little nest somewhere in the west', it was undoubtedly 'a place known to God alone' because it could be seen only from directly above, and for anyone desirous of letting the rest of the world go by, this was spot on. The entrance was unmarked, just a gate into a field, along which one drove till motor transport could proceed no further, for it was as if one had suddenly come to the edge of the world. From there, far below down the steep hillside, Hillcroft could be seen. It comprised a thatched cottage and a few farm buildings, several with their roofs falling in. If you didn't need running water, electricity, easy access or even a standard toilet, then Hillcroft might serve, but as a place to farm and earn a living it was tough going.

The new owners had spotted me descending the hill, carrying what I thought I might need. They had asked me to come and inspect their livestock, give it all the once-over and advise them on a few points, and they welcomed me as they might some long-lost uncle bearing tidings of good fortune. I thought it likely I was the first human being they had seen for some time. I was ushered into the sitting-room and there regaled with coffee right away.

'You must excuse us not being very straight and tidy, but we haven't had time to get all the things we want, and well' ... she paused ... 'we thought it more important to get some animals than a lot of furniture.' I thought they both, Mr and Mrs Robens, looked ridiculously young, the dew of innocence still upon them, and somehow very vulnerable in this big old world – and in the farming world too, which had its share of sharks swimming around looking for easy prey.

'Sorry to disappoint you,' I grinned. 'Tell me, what did you think?'

'We thought you might be older, and be big and broad, and maybe even wear a kilt.'

'A kilt in Devon?' I laughed. 'With the breezes whipping in from the Channel? As for the rest, well' (I was using it now), 'I'm big and lean instead.'

'Oh, but we're not at all disappointed,' she rushed on, 'we like you and I'm sure you will be very good.'

'That remains to be seen. Thanks for the coffee; now for some work. What do you want me to do?'

'We want you to look at all our animals and see if they are healthy, and . . . well, we want you to tell us which of our cows are going to have a calf, and when to send for the . . . man that brings the bull.' She blushed.

'You mean the artificial inseminator, AI for short. Right, we'll see the cows first.'

'We don't know very much, but I've been studying this book' (her husband waved a slim volume entitled *Farming Made Easy*), 'and we listen to "The Archers".'

'My hat,' I thought, 'innocents abroad!'

'But before you do anything, we, well, we . . . how much do you charge, and how soon do we, well, have to pay you? We could give you something today, but it might not be enough.'

That was the first time anybody had offered me money before I'd done a job, I thought. I liked them all the more!

'We send out our statements monthly, but let's forget about payment for a while until we see how you are getting on. If you need advice, you can ring me any time if you think I can help. We don't charge for phone advice.'

I could see the young fellow sigh as if a great weight had been taken from his shoulders concerning payment, and with that we headed in procession to their little cowshed, Mr

'I want to be able to tell you which cows are in calf, which are not, and how far on the pregnant ones are.'

Her face cleared. 'Oh, I see; it's just like an enema before an operation, you are doing.'

'Pardon?' I queried, not following the drift of her thought.

'I had an operation once, and I had an enema before it, but your way is much quicker and not so messy.' I stared in bewilderment, as she asked, 'But why do they need an enema before a pregnancy test?'

'I'm not really giving them an enema, Mrs Robens, it's just that you can't put your arm in a cow's rectum without getting it dirty!'

That settled, I turned again to the patiently waiting number 3. I was busy palpating the uterus when the voice came back at me again.

'But why do you need to, well, do that, and get your arm dirty? What's it for?'

'To find out if the cow is in calf or not. You can mark the first two down as not in calf.'

I could see two puzzled faces staring at me. Very slowly Mrs Robens laid down her book. I could not think what I'd said or done, but clearly their faith in Scots vets in general and this one in particular was shaken.

'But . . . but . . . you're in the wrong place,' she expostulated, while her husband blushed crimson. Then she went on, doubtfully, 'Or are cows different from people?'

I could see I had been taking too much for granted. They couldn't have heard the episode from 'The Archers' dealing with pregnancy tests. I really had to turn away from these two intent young faces to avoid doubling up in mirth. I gulped a few times, and then explained: 'The only way I can tell how far on in calf any cow may be is to examine the womb through the rectal wall. I don't go through it,' I hastened to add, before they conjured up pictures of holes poked through rectal walls. 'The womb lies below the pine, and felt that somehow our lines were crossed again.

'Show me the pine,' I demanded, peering more closely at the sheep.

'It's in the house. We keep it in the kitchen.'

'In the kitchen?'

'Yes, I've six of it.'

'Six, in the kitchen? Isn't it a bit crowded?'

'Well, the kitchen is rather small, but they only take up a little corner on a shelf,' she said, as if that made everything clear.

'I think we must be talking about different things,' I suggested. 'Pine to me is a disease – really a deficiency . . . in sheep. What is it to you?'

'Oh, I thought you meant the disinfectant which was recommended to us as fine and strong.'

That settled, I explained that pine in sheep is a disease where the sheep simply pine or waste away, and that it is the result of a deficiency of cobalt in the bloodstream, which deficiency in turn comes from the ground. I went on to explain that you could dress the ground, which was not always easy, or wholly satisfactory; the better way, certainly for the owners of six ewes, was to give the sheep, individually, a supply of cobalt.

'It's not absolutely certain that it is cobalt alone that is missing, since it has been shown that iron also, if deficient, can cause the condition. There's very little pine in Devon, but along this plateau, it occurs. I've some pellets in the car – they're called "bullets" in this case – so if you come along with me, Mr Robens, I'll let you have a supply. You can also borrow my gun for shooting them over the sheep's throats, which might save you a scratch or two. Oh, by the way, pine also occurs in cattle, so I'd dose them as well.'

Mrs Robens had been busy scribbling all this down, obviously as an appendix to *Farming Made Easy*. I could

That would give you milk, beef, eggs and pig weaners to sell, so you will always have the till ticking over.' I leapt to my feet. 'I really must be on my way.'

Accompanied by the young fellow and cheered on my way by fervent thanks from his wife, I reached the car, gave him the mineral bullets and gun, and was off. My ego had been considerably boosted because they had hung on every word I'd said, whereas in Ayrshire I was more often than not told by the farmer what he wanted, like issuing instructions to the plumber to fix a new washer on a tap.

My next call was to another 'townie' couple, who had been clients for several years now. I stopped the car at the top of their road as I always did, and gazed at one of the loveliest little bays I know – Forest Bay – which looked exactly as it sounded. At the foot the sea, surging ceaselessly in to the shore, met the forest, whose feet were almost in the waves, and whose trees covered all the visible land around, presenting a scene of great beauty and an atmosphere of timelessness. I felt I must get a photograph, for that day the sea was a deep, deep blue, contrasting with the softer blue of the sky and the various shades of green of the forest. Below, on a little knoll above the beach, stood the old manor house, looking, as always, perfect in that setting, as if it had grown up naturally with the trees. Only one thing marred the scene. Just above the tree-line, and indeed cutting into the forest itself, was a great gash of turned-up earth, a strip completely devoid of vegetation. Here stood a pig farm, a large one now, owned and run by the Ingravilles, the tenants of the Manor. I nosed the car down towards the piggery, saw no one about, and drove on down to the house.

I remembered my first visit there and my introduction to Mr Ingraville, clearly not his original name, for he was Polish and had been a cavalry officer when the Nazis invaded his homeland. His wife – well, I don't know what

'Has he been ill?' I asked.

'No, he has not,' came the raging reply, 'he has been killed – by him!' And she pointed dramatically at the wretched Walters. Lady Macbeth couldn't have done it better. Mr Ingraville meantime was spluttering in Polish, of which language I knew not a word, but I could make a very fair guess at what he was saying; just to make it clear, he ended with an explosive, 'Blast you, you murderer!'

'I tell you, I did nothing, sir. I just found him lying here,' said poor Walters.

'Pshaw – a likely story. He was quite all right an hour ago,' said Mrs Ingraville.

'We've seen you kick the boar, you wretched asass . . . asass . . . killer,' came Mr Ingraville, on cue with his line.

It was a rather nasty situation, and while I didn't go overboard for either Ingraville, neither did I think very highly of Walters. It was clear I was going to have to arbitrate in the affair, to be the detective who was to ferret out the truth. So from a veterinary surgeon who had come to discuss scouring pigs, I was changed in a moment to the pathologist in a homicide . . . or rather a pigicide. I hadn't come prepared to do a post-mortem, but I had a few scalpels in my bag, so got to work. I found the cause of death, too, to my great surprise and relief, though I doubted if it was going to help to restore normal relations and general bonhomie between the warring factions. The boar had bled to death from an internal haemorrhage in the abdomen. It could conceivably have been a kick, it could have been a fall. I could see no trace of an aneurism, and I was pretty sure in my own mind that somebody or something had landed the poor old boar a hefty thump. I explained this to the watching threesome, and immediately Mrs Ingraville went into her pointing routine with quite a long speech, the gist of which was that they would sue Walters for damages, and he was to be gone and never darken their pighouse door again.

jumping up and down in their liturgy, who burnt candles . . . even incense . . . and who bowed to the altar – all things that were utterly alien to me; yet amongst those folks, so very different from me in the expression of their faith, were men and women who were truly saintly. It was not a 'halo round the head' kind of saintliness, it was certainly not a sickly or weak thing . . . it was as if these people, from every walk of life, had learned a great secret, discovered a truth long sought . . . and found abundant wealth. They were gentle folks, and in contact with them, some of the sharp corners of my square Presbyterian position were smoothed over. The person I saw most was Ursula (Bernard could never get her name right and called her 'Hiroshima'). Ursula was in charge of the cattle and was not unlike her Guernseys, a sort of golden glow surrounding her, as if a light was burning within. But she was far from other-worldly, was an expert with cattle, and, slim little thing though she was, could tackle heavy tasks. She also had probably the cleanest, most sterile cowshed and dairy in Devon. The task for the day was simply to wash out a cow, that is, to insert a metal catheter into the womb and pump in some antiseptic solution, to clear up the lingering metritis or inflammation. But veterinary practice is full of surprises, and one often hears the words, 'Oh, when you're here anyway, would you look at such-and-such?'

The such-and-such on this occasion was a cow with an enormous lump, about the dimension of a size 3 football I used to kick as a laddie. It was one of those cases that looks much worse than it is, though I don't suppose the bearer of the lump would agree. The lump was on the chest wall, just behind the shoulder, and was in fact an abscess, probably caused by a horn-poke from another cow. This one was ripe for the knife, so having obtained an old bucket from Ursula, and advising her to stand well back and hold her nose, I lanced it, to let an enormous quantity of pus drain into the

The next call wouldn't take long, I thought. Further along to the next village, and now at the furthest point of the practice, perhaps twenty-eight miles from home, I had simply to give a dog its distemper inoculation. I found the house with difficulty, and was conducted to an upstairs flat by the landlady. I thought I was back with the dogs again, because that room stank of a mixture of cooking, stale tobacco smoke, spirits and just plain dirt. A figure rose from a couch as I entered, the landlady having simply, and without apology, thrown open the door.

'Mr Leighton-Jones?' I asked.

'Flight-Lieutenant Leighton-Jones, old boy,' came the correction.

The room was very dim, with drawn curtains, and as he switched on the light I saw a swaying form, clutching a glass in one hand and a cigarette in the other; but what instantly drew my eyes was his face. I had seen burned faces before, but none quite so dreadful as this one, which looked as if the surgeon who had done the skin-grafting had been tackling his first case.

'I'm sorry,' I said, 'I didn't know you were in the Raf.'

'Not any more, old chap . . . not any more . . . hic . . . when you're no more use to them, you're O-U-T . . . *out* . . . damn them!' he cursed.

'Were you Fighter or Bomber Command?' I inquired.

'Fighter . . . old Spitfires . . . I was one of the Few, as they called us . . . till I bought this,' he said, lifting his chin to reveal even more scarring on his neck. 'A Messerschmitt 109 got me on my tail. Pretty, isn't it . . . well, say something, damn you!' and he thrust his face close to mine. He reeked of gin, and his eyes had the bloodshot look of the heavy drinker.

I drew back involuntarily, and said simply, 'I'm very sorry.'

'Sorry! That's all we get now, sorry, sorry, sorry. What

He got up and lurched towards me, and grasped my jacket lapels. He had a point to make, it seemed, and I was his prisoner.

'By the way, what do they call you ... vet ... vet ... vet'nary surgeon, what were you with in the last show, eh? Bet it was something safe, like the Pay Corps – or no,' he paused and laughed as at some huge joke, 'it would be the Medical Corps. Half of that lot were blasted vets, I always said.'

I told him I had been too young to join up at the outbreak of war, and by the time I was that age, it was well on the way to being won; and as a vet student, I was deferred.

He sneered, gave me the full flavour of his aromatic breath, and muttered, clutching my lapels firmly, 'Knew what you were doing, eh, didn't you?'

I counted ten, laid down my case, disengaged myself from his clutch and said, 'Flight-Lieutenant, it so happened I wanted to be a vet. I am truly sorry for what you have suffered,' I held up my hand, 'though I know you don't want pity. We all in Britain owe you fellows a tremendous lot ... and we know it. But I didn't think any Battle of Britain pilot would let any Nazi fighter down him for life. If you're not a phoney, get up and fight, sir, and as for love, just look into your dog's eyes. Maybe somewhere there's another pair of eyes that still look like that, for you. Good-day to you.'

And I left him, open-mouthed, swaying on his feet. It was unfair, I thought as I left, that I who had suffered nothing should preach at someone who'd been through the hell men make of their world. It was ugly, as all cruelty is ugly – the cruelty of war, the cruelty of what it could do to people's lives – but I consoled myself with the thought of that Irish setter, to whom its master was the fairest thing on earth.

I turned the car's nose towards home with an unpleasant taste in my mouth, thinking of the callousness of that shepherd towards his dogs, and the senselessness of war that picked it up when she was dry, and unless the beast is really ill with it, and some are, very, you wouldn't notice it. We recommend that when you're drying off a cow at the end of a lactation, you fill the udder with penicillin, then seal off the teats with something like collodion. It isn't a hundred per cent, but it's as good as we know . . . that, and inoculation against it, which isn't a hundred per cent either. I'm afraid there's nothing I can do for that quarter, but she can go through life on three wheels.'

'Typical of you fellows; nowt I can do for it, then a whackin' great account.'

'Uh . . . huh . . . well, about your account, Mr Pike, we haven't had a penny for three years. I'm afraid I'll need to ask you to let us have something on account now.'

His face cleared like a summer storm passing. In so far as it was possible for Pike to become all sweetness and light, he did. He even attempted a smile, but since it was so long since he'd used the smile muscles, it came out as a kind of twisted leer.

'I know, Mr Cameron, but things have been hard lately. I'll let you have it within a fortnight.'

I looked at him suspiciously, but short of digging in my heels and saying, 'Pay now,' I didn't see what I could do, so left it at that. He even shut the car door for me as I got in, and signalled goodbye. I should have been warned!

So I turned the car homeward. It had not been a hard day; in fact in terms of numbers of visits done or difficult cases, it had been a very easy round. But in types of visit, the day had ranged from the sunshine start with those two innocent pioneers and the visit to Ursula and her Guernseys, to the encounters with the Ingravilles and Pike, the unpleasantness of the cruelty case, and the representative of the RAF . . . ex! Though few in number the visits had covered almost the whole animal spectrum, from donkey to dog. In retrospect the day had deteriorated in quality, going from good, to bad, the solar plexus to lose two large amounts. There was a certain amount of wailing and gnashing of teeth as we sought to meet our monthly drug bills, because we were at the time in one of the many financial recessions we'd experienced since 1945.

Ursula continued in her own competent way, while the Robens – well! I was wakened one morning about six-thirty by the insistent ringing of the phone. Milk fever, I thought, as I reached for it. The voice at the other end was plaintive, even accusing, and the gist of the message was that the cow I had said was seven months in calf had been due by Mrs Robens's calculations to calve that night, and, well, they had sat up all night, and it hadn't calved.

I groaned and smiled at one and the same time – which is not as easy as it sounds – and explained: 'Mrs Robens, I told you that our tests were not a hundred per cent accurate, certainly not to the day, and even if they were, cows – like people – can be ten days before or after the nine months and that is still normal.' Quite a speech for the time of day, I thought!

The client wasn't satisfied, and asked, 'But how will we know if she's calving?'

I groaned again, this time without the smile. 'Where is the cow?' I asked.

'In its shed.'

'Is it standing with its back arched, or paddling about uncomfortably on its feet, is it groaning, grunting or making any other noise, and has it any water or other discharge coming away?' – a ten-second lecture on calving.

'Well – no.'

'What is she doing?'

'Lying down and chewing her cud.'

'Then, lassie, you go and do the same – well, lie down anyway!'

The little woman phoned a week later (at a respectable

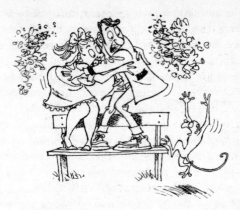

12

Monkey Tricks

I had done it! I had actually bowled an off-break. The first time I'd been a bit doubtful, thinking maybe the ball had hit a bit of dirt or something, but two in a row surely couldn't be luck. I saw myself as the Jim Laker of our Monday night team; far better to use the head and by sheer skill trap a batsman than rush up with a full head of steam, as was my wont, and find my fastest ball despatched for four. So in a state approaching bliss, I prepared to bowl a third spinner in the portion of yard at the kennels ideal for such practice, when Janet's voice summoned me back to reality. I remember there was a note of urgency in it that perfect late summer evening as she called, 'Visit, darling. Mr Trevelyan is on the phone and he seems very upset. He wants to speak to you.'

So with a sigh I threw down the ball, dreams of glory banished for the moment as I picked up the phone.

'Alex?' (in Devon they always sounded the 'x' in my name

common, most popular and certainly most mischievous of all the macaques. Many a visitor had required placating after an arm had reached out and removed his spectacles, pulled his child's hair or stolen an ice lolly. The daily cleaning of their pen was a comedy turn, for invariably one of the bunch would steal a mop or throw a bucket of water over the attendant – and now eight of these bundles of trouble were free amidst an unsuspecting public, only one of their number remaining blissfully asleep through it all, and no doubt cursing herself later that she'd missed all the fun. Three were recaptured that day, leaving five at large, in the midst of the holiday season! Of course the police had to be notified, the local paper gave wide coverage to the 'great escape', and the media kept the world informed of developments. Anyone seeing the escapees was asked to contact the zoo and for days it was inundated with calls, not one of which proved accurate. It seemed as if every dog or cat crossing a road had become a rhesus monkey, and sightings were reported from far and near. After three days a further three monkeys were captured just a mile from their home, leaving two still 'gone away'. A lady in the town found herself confronted by one of them in her hall one day. The monkey fled upstairs and went into the bathroom, whereupon the lady shut the door on it and phoned the zoo. Charlie and Irene arrived with net and box, and opened the bathroom door in time to see the monkey coolly unlatch the window and escape. However, its freedom was shortlived as it was caught the same day in a garden shed at the same house. One left to catch, but that one was to cause many heart flutterings, produce a considerable furore, and generally become a legend. Never had Bristacombe gained so much publicity, rivalling for a time Loch Ness and its famous beast! Stories abounded of the antics of this rhesus; some were no doubt apocryphal, but others had a grain of truth in them, for he was at large for weeks, enjoying to the but, causing a miniature tidal wave, she had leapt for a bath towel, with a yell that startled all her guests.

I liked the story of the little lad who had gone into the kitchen to find the monkey sitting on the table eating a banana. He rushed to the living-room and announced: 'There's a monkey on the table,' to be told not to be ridiculous. Shortly afterwards the mother had cause to go to the kitchen, and the crash of her fainting on the floor fetched her husband at the double. The monkey had by now escaped. 'I told you there was a monkey here,' Junior protested, and earned himself a hearty clout on the ear, as if he somehow had been the cause of the mother's condition. There was a state of unease around Montpellier Terrace and adjacent streets, but all efforts by Charlie and his staff to capture the errant one had been in vain. By the time they reached a sighting, the Dead End Kid was probably in another kitchen, and the uneasiness grew. A warm, well-fed monkey was probably harmless, but this one had been at large for weeks now, the nights were getting chill, and who could say what might happen?

There was one final happening, the truth of which I cannot verify, but it's a good story anyway. It concerned Billy Biddlecombe. Now the town of Bristacombe had few real drunks, but Billy was one of them, a regular soak, unless his wife kept him under restraint. On this occasion he was on his own as his wife was staying the night at South Molton with her mother, so Billy had a night out with the boys. Returning late, he fell into bed, placing the remains of a bottle of Scotch on the bedside table for night-time emergencies. Wakening late in the night, just as dawn was streaking the sky with pink fingers, Billy had felt in need of a thirst-quencher. He reached out a hand and failed to make contact with a bottle. He groped about, muttering to himself, until he became aware of other mutterings in the bedroom. His bleary eyes searched the room in vain till patience with them and made allowances for them, it was this man. He didn't miss. The little animal came cascading down the roof and its reluctant executioner had to turn away, his hands over his ears so as not to hear the thud of its fall.

I was still mystified about why I had been called by the time I reached Charlie's living-room, though desperately sorry for him. There lay the little creature beside the sack into which it had been thrown after its death. I looked at it in pity, and with interest. I had often read in Western epics of some bad lad having a hole neatly drilled between his eyes. Here I witnessed it for the first time; the hole was exactly that. I looked again.

'Charlie! He's still alive!'

I looked round at the poor man, who could only nod. Tears were coursing down his cheeks.

'Yes, Alex!' he managed to say at last. 'I want you to save him.'

I examined the monkey; it was deeply unconscious. A superficial examination failed to detect any broken ribs, but only an X-ray would show that, and who knew what internal injuries there might be – besides a bullet through the brain.

I took Charlie by the arm, made him sit down on a couch, and sat beside him.

'Now look, Charlie! You know I'm just about as fond of animals as you are, but it would take a brain surgeon to save him, and there are no vet brain surgeons. Besides, no human surgeon would attempt anything without sophisticated tests, and possibly the nearest place for that might be London. The only reason I can think of that he's not dead is that, at the angle you shot him, the bullet must have travelled upwards and missed any vital centre – but Charlie, there's only one hole. The bullet is still in there. I can't save him.'

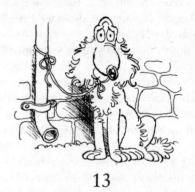

13

To Die or Let Live

Leaving the car in the private parking space of The Willows,
I quietly opened the fine wrought-iron gate which, like
everything at The Willows, betokened excellent taste and
the money to indulge it. I climbed the first few steps that led
to the garden path, as I had done often before, but today,
before proceeding any further, I paused and sat down on the
garden wall. It was quiet there, and I felt badly in need of a
few moments by myself to control my emotions before going
on to the next case. Glancing over my shoulder, I could just
see the roof of the house, and towering above it, the rocky
knoll at whose feet it nestled. Safe in the knowledge that my
presence was as yet undetected, I gave myself up to the
luxury of a rest and reflection.

It was a glorious summer day, and in the garden behind
me bees droned and buzzed as they inspected the many
flowers for nectar, while in the shrubs and trees blackbirds
sang, sparrows chirruped and chaffinches chattered. In

these ponies. Two weeks ago he had been with them, someone on his back, probably a child experiencing the thrill of a first riding lesson, for Silver was quiet, gentle, trustworthy, ideal for beginners – and just two streets away from The Willows, Silver was dying in the loosebox where I'd left him.

It had been perhaps ten days ago that John Wilkinson, owner of the stables, had called me. Silver had been brought in with the other ponies to be groomed and made ready for another day's toil over the dunes, and up the hill and fields beyond. But something was clearly wrong with the little grey pony that morning. He walked stiffly, dragging behind the others, and stood in his box listless, head down, pained-looking. Silver had a temperature and I set out to discover why.

'He was all right yesterday, and when we put them out to grass last night,' said his owner, as I listened to Silver's chest with my stethoscope. His lungs were clear, though his respirations were faster than normal. He had no nasal discharge, no obvious abscesses, just that stiff, 'don't want to move' look. What was it? I ran my hands over neck, back and limbs – nothing. It was only when I ducked under his head at the feeding trough that I found it, and as soon as I touched his brisket (the pad of muscle and fat at the front of the chest), he whinnied and reared. The wound there was not big, but already it was a dirty, almost black, colour. I didn't like it, for I knew what had caused that wound, or was at any rate ninety-nine per cent certain – an adder. Every summer we had adder bites. Every summer I'd treated cattle and sheep, but principally dogs, and all had recovered uneventfully. I'd never seen one in a horse, and by the look of it that wound had happened the night before, probably just after he'd been turned out to grass and had lain down for a roll and a delicious scratching of the back to get all the itchiness and stiffness out of him. He must have lain on the

The Willows. Even now the inspector would be on his way; perhaps already he'd arrived, and soon there would be a merciful release. I blamed myself for not finishing the job, and puzzled again if there was more I could have done; one always did. These moments communing with Nature didn't take away the disappointment, but they brought some healing and put things in perspective. The tides would still ebb and flow, birds would still sing, and up in these dunes a few adders would still lurk for the unwary like the gentle Silver, for the ceaseless war in Nature of creature upon creature, and the constant fight to counteract the evil, would still be ours to win or lose.

At last I went on up to the villa, one of several in that lofty place. I'm sure the gardens were a blaze of glory – they always were at The Willows – but they were passed unnoticed that afternoon. I rang the front-door bell and Miss Plumtree and a horde of dogs answered the call. I knew that there were, in fact, eight dogs, all cocker spaniels. I wasn't too clear about the number of Plumtree sisters. There were three I'd met at their fine house with its magnificent view, while others were vaguely alluded to, but the number of dogs was always eight. The sisters were aged anything from fifty to seventy-five; it was impossible to say, for they dressed, wore their hair and conversed in a way that was pure Victoriana. The furniture of the house and the jungle of pot plants in every room all spoke of a bygone age. Clearly the sisters had been well endowed by father Plumtree, long since deceased, but despite their wealth they always seemed to me rather forlorn, left behind like driftwood on the beach when the tide has ebbed, and a little bemused by this strange modern world. They were called Emily, Letitia and Victoria, and in the way they fluttered around, fussed, became flustered, yet always remained completely courteous, I thought I could see Miss Marple, Agatha Christie's famous detective with the kindly manner but air of bewilderment.

'And that man Attlee. It beats me how dear Winston can possibly stand him,' she went on.

I am a strictly non-political animal, certainly in public, but I was moved to say, 'Oh, I don't know, Miss Plumtree. He did a lot during the war, and he and Mr Churchill seemed to work well together then.'

'But he's such a *little* man . . . and as for the rest of his gang . . .' She left it unsaid, but I had a picture of Messrs Wilson, Dalton, Bevan and their colleagues with masks on their faces and bags marked 'Swag' on their backs. I hastily changed the subject.

'These are lovely scones, Miss Plumtree. Who's the baking expert?'

'Our Mrs Buxton does most of it, but these are actually Emily's.'

Little Emily looked abashed, embarrassed but also pleased. I fancy nobody ever took notice of poor Miss Emily. The meal proceeded to its leisurely close, the trays were removed, then Miss Victoria leaned back to issue the order of the day.

'It's little Rupert. We want you to take him away and put him to sleep.'

I gasped! 'But he's only a baby. It's only months since I gave him his distemper inoculation.' I looked at Rupert lying peacefully on a couch. 'What on earth's wrong with him?'

'His ears are too long for a cocker; they get in his food and this will certainly lead to ear canker. Also he's had one or two little cysts between his toes. I'm afraid he's from a weakly strain.'

'But, Miss Plumtree, ear canker and interdigital cysts are nothing, and can be easily treated. You can't put a dog down for that.' Attempting to be flippant, I added, 'It's like putting Mr Attlee down because he's too small!'

'And a very good thing too.' Clearly I'd said the wrong thing. She went on, 'But it's a totally different matter.

only with a clear conscience, but with a smile of bliss. Did Christian Scientists believe that? I must check.

So Rupert accompanied me to the car. I knew in a few weeks I would be summoned to Epivax his successor, and keep up the required number of eight. The little black dog frisked and frolicked all the way to the surgery, eagerly studying the passing scene. With our specially concentrated Euthatal, all he knew was the prick of a needle, in five seconds blissful sleep. In thirty seconds he was dead. The death sentence had been passed and carried out. I felt a bit sick.

There was another dog tied up in our back premises, also a spaniel, but this time a large dun-and-white one with brown splotches on her, and the most gentle face and tender eyes you ever saw.

'What's that one in for, Mrs Drury?' I asked.

'To be put down.'

'What! Why?'

'I'm not sure why. She's not young, she has a small mammary tumour, but I think they've just got tired of her.'

'Who were her owners?'

'I didn't know them. They were strangers to me, just paid cash and left.'

'Well, Mrs Dru, I'm not doing it. I'll take her home.'

So the dog became part of the Cameron household. The name Lass seemed to suit her, and she soon readily answered to it. She proved herself to be a lovely, quiet, soft creature, gentle with the children, beloved by them, and the most obedient member of the family! The tumour was tiny, benign, harmless. One day I'd remove it, but there was no hurry. I don't know if Lass had any thoughts of the delights of some future life, but she most certainly enjoyed her remaining time in this one. She was one of those where the decision was to let live, to the delight of all concerned.

At nine that evening the phone rang. Janet and I looked at

here, I'll oblige, though matted hair is common in old cats and can be cut off or combed out. Besides, I was on your farm just the other day, and no mention was made of it then. Surely it hasn't grown old in a matter of days?'

Long pause . . . I guessed what was coming. Still very polite . . .

'Oh, Mr Cameron, brother and I were talking one night and we thought it might be an advantage to have two veterinary surgeons, from different practices. If you don't feel you can come tonight, I might have to ring someone else.'

He'd come this blackmail once before and had insisted I turn out quite late one evening to see a lame ram, which he admitted had been lame for nearly a week but which definitely needed treatment that evening. Not wanting to antagonize a client, I had successively bitten my lip, gnashed my teeth, frothed at the mouth, and gone. But not tonight. I'd had enough killing for one day. So, equally politely, I replied, 'Well, now, Mr Parkhurst, that might be a very good idea and then you could ring your other vet alternate Fridays for advice. Yes, a good idea! But if you do decide you still want my services, you can give me a ring in the morning or bring the cat in tomorrow, for it's getting a bit late to come tonight. Good-night to you!'

I slammed down the phone in great glee. I'd wanted to do that for a long time to old Parkhurst . . . the man who paid his bills to us once a year and then asked for discount . . . the man who kept his bills to a minimum by regular free advice by phone . . . the farmer who usually didn't want you to call unless you were passing anyway, so that he wouldn't have to pay a visit fee, but who expected instant service when he clapped his hands. Yes, I'd enjoyed that. There was a lot of the unregenerate in me yet!

Parkhurst was at the surgery next morning, cat-basket in one hand, a jar of cream as a peace offering in the other. I

I have since then, over many years and almost weekly, stood beside a bed and watched someone fight a brave but losing battle, and I've pondered deeply. It is my view that in such cases, assuming everything is being done to ease the patient's suffering, to take life would be, very often, to deprive a husband or wife of experiences and moments that are very precious and forged only in the fires of suffering, shared together. But there are other cases where I've wondered . . . I have gone into an enormous ward of geriatric patients, the beds close together, scarcely allowing passage between them, beds containing people who have lost all awareness of surroundings and all control of their actions; I have seen folks lose all dignity, privacy, individuality, and become increasingly distressing for their loved ones to behold week by week. Cabbages! That's how society has labelled such poor beings. I know all the arguments against any form of euthanasia, at any time, and respect deeply the views of all who hold them. I have the highest regard for the sanctity of human life, and a deep love of old folks. As a minister of the Gospel, I have no doubts of the reality of that other world, nor of our basic belief that man is an eternal spirit. I know all the questions regarding any form of euthanasia – I give no answers. I only know that many times I've come away from a scene of extreme weakness or debility, and with indignation and concern have said to myself, 'I wouldn't treat a dog like that!' I have, conscious (oh, so conscious) of my own helplessness, wondered what He, who was and is far from helpless, and whose hands in Galilee were tender to soothe and to save, would do in our day, in a ward of folks weary, longing, sighing, yes! and asking to be released to 'go home' – and I've heard an echo as of old, saying, 'Blessed are the merciful – for they shall obtain mercy.'

Fardley was one of these little out-of-the-way places that abound in Devon and are part of its charm. I felt my spirits rise as I drove along and a song came to my lips. (One of our students seeing practice had once reported to his wife in wonderment, 'He sings as he drives!') It was a gorgeous May morning, fields were greening up with early summer freshness, trees were bursting into leaf, birds were skimming merrily in front of the little Austin van as she cruised along the famous sunken Devon lanes. They weren't really sunken. It was simply that generations of farmers had built dykes, then covered them with earth, and on top planted a hedge, thus making high walls which were excellent windbreaks from the cold nor'-easterlies or wet westerlies for sheep and out-wintered cattle. These were the high hedges that had driven my old teacher Sandy Gray to distraction on his honeymoon years ago in Devon, when he snorted, 'Glorious Devon, if you could see anything over these hedges!' – a sentiment that many had echoed since. But it was glorious Devon that morning, with the high banks a mass of yellow primroses. Yes, it was good to be alive, to be free, to be a country vet on such a day, so why not sing a stave or two! I had been through Fardley before, a tiny hamlet tucked away off the main roads, just a cluster of houses and little farms, and a sign marked 'Post Office' pointing vaguely in the direction of a small thatched house. Roses were already in bloom on the walls, lupins and peonies making splashes of colour in the borders, as I walked up the path and entered.

I had apparently been observed, for there behind a tiny counter was a little old lady with rosy cheeks, eyes creased with wrinkles which I suspected had been produced more by smiles than tears, and a gentleness and serenity about her. She greeted me with a hearty 'Good-morning' and equally heartily I agreed it was, and asked if she could direct me to the Grange.

explained the little wife. 'She's Chapel, like us; we're mostly Chapel hereabouts; it's Grizelda,' she added. I wasn't sure whether that lady was also Chapel, but thought it was about time I saw her. First, however, Mr Hopkins had to explain.

'We've mostly had Mr Warman before' (Warman was the opposition – a deadly and not always very ethical rival), 'but you're just as near, and we heard you were Scottish and the Scottish were very good with cattle.' I thought wryly that we used to have a great name for stealing English cattle – but hoped I would live up to their expectations; nevertheless, a cow with a stroke could mean anything from a cerebral haemorrhage to a tumour on the brain.

Eventually I was allowed to see Grizelda, little Mrs Hopkins bounding on in front and throwing open the door of a loose-box. In one corner was a calf some twenty-four hours old, while on a deep bed of spotlessly clean straw lay Grizelda, deeply unconscious. I tested her eye and ear reflexes, took her temperature and pulse, my every move being watched intently. I felt I must go through the motions and justify their faith in Scots vets – but one glance would have told the most raw recruit to the veterinary profession, even if he hadn't the initial advantage of a Scots pedigree, what was what. I had been astonished since coming to Devon at the many who had not seen a condition that was a daily occurrence back in Ayrshire, and in most dairying districts of Britain.

'Never had aught like this before,' boomed Mr Hopkins, as if divining my thought.

'Can you do anything?' earnestly entreated his little wife.

'Yes, Mrs Hopkins, I think I can soon put Grizelda right. Could you just bring me a bucket of water, not too hot, soap and a towel?'

She departed at the double while I got out my flutter-valve, calcium bottles, tin of needles, bottle of iodine and a swab. Then, having put one of the calcium bottles in the

the hour lurched to her feet unsteadily and headed for her calf who was giving tongue from one corner, while farmer Hopkins, on equally rubbery legs, staggered up from the other. They were like two punch-drunk boxers who'd had about enough. Little Mrs Hopkins was ecstatic, and hopped about betwixt one and the other, enthusing, 'My, sir, it's just like the Bible – Lazarus being raised from the dead, or being born over again!'

I didn't know whether she was referring to her husband or Grizelda, though I fancied the latter, and agreed it was a good description. Over the inevitable cup of tea, which I waited to drink to make sure the old man was all right (one was offered tea at virtually every call in North Devon), I explained the phenomenon to them.

'Your cow had milk fever, Mr Hopkins. In the old days they thought it was a germ in the milk that caused it, so it got the name, and they used to inject a weak solution of iodine into the udder – mighty uncomfortable, but now and then it saved a cow's life. It was certainly better than the older cure of whisky, which never yet saved a cow with milk fever, but I suppose by the time the cow had had a drink, and the farmer and the vet a few each, they were all past caring anyway when the poor beast died. By and by somebody on the Continent found that you didn't need iodine, that water would do; then somebody again found that to pump the udder up with air was even better. But all these were shots in the dark. When they worked, it was simply because they stopped the udder producing milk, which allowed the level of calcium in the cow's blood to rise again, but of course the udder was often ruined. Then in the 1930s a Scots vet' (I had to get in a plug and keep up their regard for our ability) 'took blood tests from a hundred cows suffering from milk fever. In every case the blood-calcium level was too low, so what we do now is simply inject calcium. Mind you,' I went on with utter sincerity, 'I've seen this hundreds of times and it was only fastened at one end, so that the other stuck out in front like a direction-finder.

'Quite extraordinary!' he announced. (He certainly was, but I don't think he meant it autobiographically.) 'Oh, hello, Mrs Hopkins – Percival, good-day to you,' he said, proceeding to raise a hat, then finding there was none there. He tried to fasten his clerical collar to its retaining stud and appear presentable. I gazed fascinated as the collar-end came away again with a 'Ping!'. The poor man grabbed it in one hand and me in the other.

'Look here, Mr . . . er . . . er . . . Cameron. I put a call through to my own vet, Mr Darnaway' (I didn't mind him; he was a cheerful old chap, and co-operative, unlike the vindictive Warman), 'but he is out on a case; then I telephoned you, to discover you were actually here in Fardley. It seemed quite providential, but whether you can do anything, I doubt. The poor animal seems stark, raving mad.' 'Ping!' went his collar yet again, as he tried in vain to fasten it with one hand.

'Is it a cow, or a bull, or a young beast?' I inquired.

'It's a two-year-old heifer,' he explained as he led me to his shippen – his recalcitrant collar periodically pinging merrily as he led me on.

'See, in here,' he whispered, lest the mad beast would hear us, and he peeped in the top half of the stable-type door. 'Quite, quite gone,' he said, pointing to his head. It wasn't clear whether he meant himself or his heifer, it being a moot point which was looking the wilder, but I gave him the benefit of the doubt. 'Have you ever seen anything like that before?' he demanded.

'Yes, a few times, but this one's a beaut!'

'Really.' He paused, and further exclaimed, 'Extraordinary!', as if it was beyond the realms of understanding that there should be so many mad bovines in the world. Then he asked rather piteously, poor man, 'Can anything be done?'

'Then, Vicar . . . ah . . . Rector, if you have a rope handy we'll prepare for a heavenly visitation.' He looked at me doubtfully. Did I seem too flippant, I wondered? I hastily went on to explain.

'We have no hope unless we can restrain that heifer somehow, and what better way than from above? Now, I'll go up into the hayloft and drop a noose over her head. When she charges she'll pull the slip knot tight, and it's up to you and Mr Hopkins here to get in beside her and secure her by that rope to a post, stanchion, anything. It'll be hot work . . . maybe you should take your collar off.'

So the pinging collar ceased to ping, but there followed an equally mad fifteen minutes. Several times I had the dangling noose almost over the beast, but always she dodged. Finally I suggested the Rector should call to her over the stable half-door, and from the loft immediately above, when she headed for the door, I would try to lasso her. Thankfully, it worked, the rope pulled tight and flew out of my hands, but the big, burly farmer and the lean, rangy churchman were in there like a flash, grabbing the trailing end of the rope and securing it round a post. I swung down from my lofty abode to lend a hand. That heifer struggled like mad. I tied another rope round her horns, gradually releasing the lasso, which by now was all but throttling her.

'Now, Rector, you pray that I can hit this jugular vein pretty soon, and that the magnesium will be in time to work, but I warn you, it can also kill sometimes. Mr Hopkins, I suggest you look the other way.'

I wasn't so expert with jugular as mammary veins, having trained on Ayrshires, where the mammary vein was about an inch in diameter. However, at the third jab I got it, and once again the flutter-valve routine was repeated, but this time much more slowly, as I watched the respiratory rate with care. The beast quietened a bit, its flutterings beneath us lessening.

animals rescued from death in quiet little Fardley that morning, thanks to medical science and a modicum of skill in the operator. So different from the poor old Rector, I thought. Apart from his glebe-land, which he farmed as part of his living, what results could he show? The thoughts passed idly through my mind, with no realization then that I would often return to these very questions in my next vocation – but more of that anon.

I've quite often noticed how you've seldom been near a place, and then suddenly you seem never to be away from it. So it was for a time with the little community of Fardley. Two weeks after their milk fever, the Hopkins had milk trouble again. This time it was reported that a sow named Jemima had farrowed a litter of fourteen – and had no milk. Could I come? I grabbed that one for myself before Bernard could volunteer, for we both especially loved that district of the practice. As the Austin headed once more for the Grange, I thought ahead, as vets do, to what was likely to await me. Almost certainly this was agalactia, which simply means, of course, no milk. Again, as with milk fever, it is a misnomer. In fact, the sow delivers her piglets, and nature provides her with a requisite number of teats and milk enough to feed her hungry brood – but something has gone wrong with the mechanism. There's a spanner in the works, an infinitesimal fault, but with disastrous results. The 'let-down hormone', as it is called, produced by the tiny pituitary gland in the brain, triggers off the mechanism – releases the trapdoor, if you like – to let the milk flow. Without that hormone functioning, the udders can be bursting with milk, to the sow's acute discomfort and the piglets' utter despair, yet not a single drop will come and the piglets will starve to death.

Two pictures always came to my mind when I thought of this condition. One was of a lecturer we had, a bumptious him he could look now, and at his expectant glance said, 'Now we wait a little. How's Grizelda?'

They took me to the little one-acre orchard where she was grazing, whistled her up to the gate, and the gentle creature stood there, placidly chewing the cud and regarding me with her big brown eyes as I stroked her head. Mrs Hopkins twittered, 'Here's Mr Cameron, Grizel – he saved your life, you know.' Grizel chewed on. Life was good now, why think of the past! The reunion over, we went back to look at mother and piglets. I knew before we reached the pen that all was well. No longer was there the squeal of hungry piglets, but instead that lovely deep baritone grunt of a sow suckling its young, while from each little knob came a contented sucking note, like a line of bellringers pulling their ropes in turn.

'Well, I do declare,' said Mrs Hopkins, 'if I didn't know you for a Chapel-goer I would say you were a wizard. Do you never fail, Mr Cameron?'

'Often,' I said. 'You just haven't found me out yet!'

I was presented with a jar of Devon clotted cream for Mrs Cameron, and pressed to take the service in their little Methodist chapel sometime. I promised I would, with pleasure, and I meant it. They were the salt of the earth, these simple, straight, homely folks.

I thought I'd have a quick call at the Rectory. I was met by the Rector in full clerical attire, just off to a diocesan meeting. 'Would you have a quick look at a lamb?' he asked. 'It's a late one,' he explained, 'and is all crippled and poorly.'

I looked at the pathetic wee beast and gave him a rapid synopsis. 'Joint ill, for certain – infection through the navel at birth, localization and swelling in the joints, either will die or won't thrive – unless you're prepared to spend something on it and a lot of time with it, and even then I can't promise.' He said he would try. He was a kindly soul, and he knew what it was to have frequent infirmities himself! So I gave the

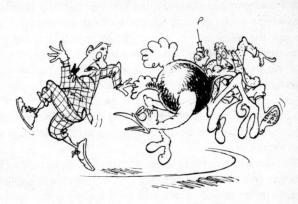

15

Variety Pack

'Bernard, what's a coypu?' I asked as I put down the phone.

'Haven't a clue,' came his prompt reply.

'I think it's like a rat, only bigger,' said Ann. We both looked at her in admiration, not only because she was easy on the eye, but regularly our new secretary would surprise us with the scope of her knowledge. Two weeks ago she'd put us right on an ocelot.

'Charlie in trouble again, then?' asked Bernard.

'Well, his coypu is. It doesn't sound very much, and if it's only a kind of rat, I reckon I can manage. If it had been those black bears, Bernard, I'd have remembered a calving in the middle of Exmoor! Besides, there are a few things he would like me to see, so I'll get a free conducted tour of the zoo – maybe if I'm in luck I'll get a choc-ice going in!'

It was a glorious warm, early summer afternoon, just the kind of sleepy day for a leisurely zoological expedition – plus a choc-ice, to which I am somewhat partial. Bernard time, as immutable now as when beasts first walked our planet – that the weakest goes to the wall. So animals, even in captivity, would often mask symptoms of illness from their fellow creatures and from man till they could hide them no more, and by then, from the vet's point of view, it was too late. Case after case could be quoted to illustrate this law of the wild.

I remember being gripped urgently by Charlie at the gate one day and rushed to the puma's cage. I knew a puma was a mountain lion and was therefore a member of the cat family, but my life hitherto had been completely puma-free, and as Charlie hustled me cagewards that day I felt that doom had come upon me. I was in mortal terror of either disgracing myself by fleeing from the cage, gibbering with terror – or by not making it to the door before the puma had sampled me! As it happened I needn't have worried, for I could see as we reached his cage that the puma was breathing his last. I reached for the adrenaline bottle, but before any stimulant could be given our patient had gone, his final gesture being a despairing lunge with one paw at us – at man, the ancient foe. I looked at that great cat lying there, and if there was – I admit – a sense of relief in my heart, there was also a feeling of great pity. He was beautiful, so sleek and graceful, even in death. I suppose he had been happy there – he had certainly been well cared for – but every sinew of his legs, his powerful hip and shoulder muscles, his proud eye, now unseeing – all had been designed for him to wander the high uplands of his homelands . . . and he had died, far away, in a cage.

'There didn't seem a thing wrong with him till yesterday, when he was a bit off colour, and then today he wouldn't eat at all,' said Charlie.

'Sure?'

'Certain sure' – and you can't be surer than that in Devon.

'Let's see then, Charlie, what killed him.'

I carried out a post-mortem there in his cage, the great

of the same ilk. The beauty of many skin conditions is that they are delightfully vague, and even for the expert, treatment is often a case of trial and error.

The coypu dealt with, Charlie took me on a conducted tour; he had time on his hands. He wanted to show me new additions and get some advice, and since I also had time I was content to wander round the whole zoo. Almost every cage, every enclosure, brought back memories of battles won or lost, and everywhere were creatures I had seen before and treated for injury or disease. First we went to the aviaries, where Charlie had about the best and biggest collection of birds in Britain at the time – hundreds of them. The overriding impression when you entered was one of colour and sound. It seemed as if some artist had been busy and made merry with every known colour. Bright reds were equalled by vivid greens; softer orange matched gentler pink, while pastel shades abounded. Over all was the chatter of sound: the screeching of parrots, the call of the mynah bird, the soft intimate murmurs of dozens of pairs of budgerigars; there were macaws, chaffinches, cockatoos, canaries, dozens of species, the noise inside being augmented from time to time by the quacking of muscovy ducks outside, the scream of a peacock or the hissing of a goose. It was here in the aviaries that I'd had my greatest failures. These birds, I soon found, are very subject to nose, throat and chest infections. I kept peering suspiciously for psittacosis, but it was always straightforward chills, croups, bronchitis, pneumonias, or so it seemed, and naturally I had used, where I thought it necessary, penicillin. I might as well have given potassium cyanide. For what reason I know not, penicillin was fatal to or useless for my avian patients. So we switched to chloromycetin, a broad-spectrum antibiotic, and it was as dramatically successful as penicillin had been lethal. We loitered long in the aviaries; you could have spent an afternoon there. Then we moved outside to the children's carrying the black bag while I carried the tray. Barclay swung the bag at the gate meaningfully, to show he was with the vet – like showing your ticket in some soccer battleground to demonstrate you are one of the combatants.

Charlie was waiting for us at the ostrich pen. Since it was Sunday, all his assistants were off-duty. I walked in and stopped dead – 'quite a big cut' was a conservative description. In fact at first sight it seemed to me it was all cut and no whole. Closer inspection showed that the ostrich had ripped its neck from top to bottom, exactly like a zip coming undone. Apparently a protruding nail had been the cause. I looked at my patient in bewilderment, and probably it showed, for Charlie reassured me that all I had to watch was his feet. I glanced down. I believed him; the ostrich's feet were bigger than my size 11s and equipped with useful-looking nails on the end of each toe. I then looked up, and realized what big birds ostriches were. I had never been this close to one before and it towered above me. I had been well instructed on how to cast or otherwise restrain horses weighing a ton and bulls weighing about fifteen hundredweight, and had proved these methods reliable many times in practice, but nobody had ever told me how to restrain this bundle of feathers weighing but a fraction of my horse or bull.

Anaesthetic, I thought, but what? I had never tried any form of general anaesthesia on birds before, and didn't think I ought to practise on the biggest of them. So, with more confidence than I was feeling, I announced, 'I'll spray the edges of the wound with this to take some of the pain away,' and proceeded to scoosh half a container of ethyl chloride on to the ostrich. Now the great thing about ethyl chloride is that you can see where it is because a layer of frost forms, but its drawback, as with all local anaesthetics, is that it only freezes the surface. To get deeper I'd need to inject all round that wound, and somehow I didn't think that was the best

'Get a sack,' I suggested. Charlie obliged – that is, once he had leapt or fallen from his mount. 'Now when he sits down again, put that over his head. It's just too bad if some dirt drops in the wound, but at least I'll maybe be able to creep up on him without being seen and make a start.'

In time, the ostrich did its celebrated flop and was blind-folded, and while I emptied the remains of my ethyl chloride spray on the wound, I commanded my assistant-acting-unpaid to return with the suture tray, which he did with the greatest reluctance and a murmured 'Oh, Mummy, Daddy . . .' over and over again, like some African incantation. Perhaps that's when the lad gained his first liking for liturgy! Whether it was the sack, the extra ethyl chloride, Barclay's spoken plea, my unspoken one – or just the sheer exhaustion of the bird. I know not, but it sat still for the remainder of the proceedings. Feeling like a seamstress who has just com-pleted a particularly long stitching stint, I inserted the last suture, packed the wound around with sulphonamide pow-der, and with Barclay safely out of the door, whipped the sack off the head. The ostrich sat on, seemingly now at peace with the world, while Charlie and I wearily made our way from its pen.

'It should be all right, I think, but you understand I've never stitched an ostrich before, so I'll look in for a couple of days to see how the wound's healing. Meantime, Charlie, for Pete's sake get a hammer and knock that nail in, so that it doesn't un-zip itself again. Come to think of it, a wee tap on the crown with a hammer might have let us get the job done more quickly. I'll remember to bring one for general anaesthetic purposes next time!'

We departed for what I felt was a well-earned tea, while Barclay went happily home with two ostrich feathers and many a tale to tell. The wound healed perfectly, and the scar was almost invisible in the flabbiness of ostrich-skin neck. As for Charlie, I don't believe he ever knocked that nail in, or was good and to the credit of his brother man (or person!). We paused a moment by the chimps, not knowing then that Bernard and he would spend a whole night trying to recapture one which had escaped and which refused point blank to re-enter its cage, and I looked at Lulu and Fifi, the star attractions of the time, totally ignorant that glorious day of the pathos that was to come for one of them – but that's another tale. So by devious routes we had come again to the main entrance gates, where, in his enclosure, a healthy, fat sea-lion was taking a cool dip. Again we paused, and again memory took us back.

'Do you remember?' Charlie began.

'Fine,' I replied.

The sea-lion was being sick, had lost weight, and was listless and generally off colour. Since sea-lions were again an untaught species at college, I contacted Oliver Jones, the famous London Zoo vet, who tried for years to breed from the giant panda at his zoo. But if he was unsuccessful in that venture, he was successful in many others, and a mine of information for the uninformed like me.

'Has he recently lost his mate?' he asked at once when I gave him the sea-lion's symptoms. I'm sure I held the phone away from my ear and looked at it in wonderment. This man was hot stuff!

'As a matter of fact he has, but how did you guess, and what's the condition?'

'Almost certainly an ulcer – peptic or possibly duodenal. I've seen it a few times here after one of our sea-lions has lost its mate. Only answer is a new mate; he's pining, anxious – typical syndrome.'

I reported the expert opinion to Charlie. That particular type of sea-lion was about £300 at the time, and Charlie, I imagine, had already overspent on other species.

'I can't possibly afford a new mate just now. Can you try something?'

rather, I should say I played a church organ. Got me £80 a year and helped to put me through college.'

'What church would that be, now?'

'Oh, a wee country church – Church of Scotland,' I said.

'Mine was a country one too – but C. of E. But Alex, when you look at a view like that, what do denominations matter? You just want to sing together, in harmony, in praise to the Almighty. You know, Alex, we can learn a lot from the animals. Look how many there are living in harmony, some of them natural enemies too. It can be done. Did you know that I once had, as the Bible says, "the lion lying down with the lamb"? They were called Leo and Persil. Word got around about them, natural enemies being great pals – of course they were both young, you understand. Anyway, I was asked to take them and any other animal to a service for animals in St Paul's, Covent Garden. Canon May took it. Went again the next year and took a monkey and Jill, an African grey parrot. She disgraced me. The Canon was a big man – weighed about eighteen stone. He had to stop for several rests·going up the pulpit stairs to get his breath. When he finally made it, Jill shouted, "Cor!" The Canon, the verger and the congregation exploded. Later in the service the Canon stopped to mop his brow, and up pipes Jill with "There's a pretty boy!" It was a good address, about being kind to God's creatures and what we could learn from them, but I was on edge with my wretched parrot. She kept butting in. When Canon May said, "Let us consider the king of the beasts," up she pipes again with "Pretty poll!" But the Canon took it all in good part. He was a fine man, gone now.'

So we sat on, reluctant to take our eyes from the view before us or shatter the peace that wrapped us round that day. I felt I would be content to live in this glorious country overlooking the Bristol Channel and tend animals there all my days, but it was decreed otherwise. Bernard remains in practice. But there is no zoo on the hill to visit; the zoo, with

PART TWO

In the Vestry

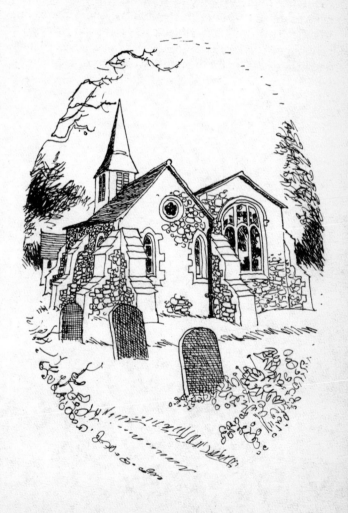

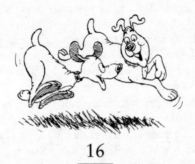

16

The Monkey on my Back

We moved into Moorton's old, large, but homely Manse a month after I had preached for the charge. It was a house that seemed to say 'Welcome' as soon as you crossed the threshold. Many generations of ministers had lived there, going back 300 years to the first, who had been ejected from this very house by a dozen dragoons on the order of the Bishop; for King Charles II, like his father and grandfather, was determined to be head of the Kirk of Scotland and impose episcopacy. After all, he reasoned, he ruled by divine right . . . But Scotland's people worshipped a higher divine, and in consequence many, like Moorton's first minister, were forced from their homes and church buildings to shelter in caves and worship behind a dyke, with their guards posted to warn of any approaching Redcoats – the guards were later to form the Cameronian Regiment. I prowled around the house, and with my love of history I felt it a tremendous privilege to be in this place, so steeped in the each spring, with the shrill call of lambs and the deeper bleat of the ewes in many a field. My fingers would start to itch, for perhaps above all I'd loved the lambing season, never ceasing to marvel at this annual miracle: the unfading wonder of delivering a lamb, saving a life, and seeing a contented mother nuzzle her lamb, while the little creature, on shaky legs but with unerring, inborn accuracy, would head straight for the source of food. Driving past fields of lambs was the hardest thing of all, but even a cat curled up on a sunlit window ledge, or a couple of dogs romping in a park, stirred the memory. Animals I loved – treating them had been not only my livelihood, but my life – and, fool that I was, I'd given it up. 'Idiot!' the monkey continually chattered in my ear. Then there was the financial side. After years of building, the practice was really taking off, and just when I could look forward to taking on another one or two colleagues, being the senior, and being comfortably off, I'd given it up. 'Madman!' said the monkey. I couldn't argue about it. From a secure future with our own house, a spare car for my wife and a considerable income, I was going into a 'tied' house, an uncertain life, for congregations could be fickle and easily tire of their minister, and all for the low salary for which most churches expected the wife to serve as well as her husband. What had I done? By every human standard the whole thing was sheer lunacy, and my decision would result in years to come in my family being denied many things they would otherwise have had.

Again the monkey had whispered (a very insidious argument this . . . he really was an intelligent ape): 'You are throwing away five hard years of study in a course infinitely more difficult than theology, years for which your parents sacrificed much for you.' That, too, was undeniable. My mother had kept hens, ducks, geese, turkeys; she had sold eggs and, every Christmas, fowls for the table, when the whole family and two old friends would sit around in a cold family, there were no university grants and, in the post-war years of depression, wages were low. There was no way he could realize his wish, so he had taken any job he could get and had become a railwayman. Moreover, he would never even see his eldest son as a minister because he had been snatched away in his fifties, just before my course commenced. I was far from clear about all the whys and wherefores of my move. In the cold light of day they didn't seem to make much sense, nor could they be explained to others. I just knew that, willy-nilly, I seemed to have been gradually propelled along this path. Kenneth, as a lay preacher, had inveigled me into it, and my involvement had grown until I was preaching every second Sunday in one or other of Devon's many little Methodist, Congregational or Baptist chapels. I'd always been keen on youngsters, and took part in different kinds of youth work. I had been taught to believe – and proved to my own satisfaction that it was true – that life's surest foundation was a sound Christian faith.

'But why did you become a minister?' Francis Gay of the *Sunday Post* once asked me on the phone. How could you cram all the forces at work, the issues involved, into a short, snappy answer on a telephone, to an unknown voice at the other end? I'd answered something like this:

'In North Devon, with its many small farms, the vet was treated very much like the family doctor, so you came to know your clients well, not just as clients, but in many cases as friends. Your advice was asked on all kinds of things, quite apart from their animals. As time went by, I came to see in this life there are really only two kinds of people – not Scots or English; rich or poor; Labour or Conservative; black or white, but those who had this strange, intangible thing we call faith, and those who hadn't. The former might not be in church every Sunday, but it seemed to me, as an outsider looking in, that this faith was very real, something that she'd married Alexander Cameron, not a vet or a minister, but the man – bless her!

So I wrestled in my study that day. The voice whispered: 'There's still time to turn back!'

If I'd been a swearing man, I would have said, 'Go to hell!', and even if this might not have been accurate geographically, it would certainly have been sound theologically concerning the wretched creature on my back. I just groaned aloud, and held my drooping head.

'Now, now,' came the voice in soft, soothing tones, 'stop worrying and fussing. You're just being prudent. You can do far more for the Christian cause as a layman than in a dog-collar. What's happened is simply the concern any person brought up in a good, devout Christian home would have for helping others, and telling others about your God. Well . . . you've just let it go to your head a bit. Besides, as a vet you would have more money to give away to charities, churches and missions. Pull out now!'

The arguments were subtle, the battle hard, but Gethsemane cannot be avoided. Tomorrow night one of the questions at ordination would be: 'Are not zeal for the glory of God, love for the Lord Jesus Christ, and a desire for the salvation of men, so far as you know your own heart, your great motives and chief inducements to enter into the office of the Holy Ministry?' No man can answer that without a clutch at the throat, and great heart-searching. But it's a question that cannot be ducked or glossed over.

So, when the family were in bed and the noises of the world were hushed, like King George VI on the night before his Coronation slipping into Westminster Abbey to be alone, I went quietly by myself into Moorton's lovely old kirk and there in the silence faced up to that question. All around me were the influences of the past. The very hush of that place seemed to carry an echo of many voices, of men and women to whom this house of prayer was the dearest

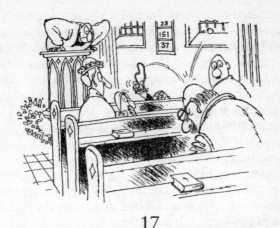

17

Welcome

'I regret to have to tell you that your new minister is not the man you think he is. In fact he has a past – quite a past. He's been in trouble with the police.'

The congregation was silenced. There were gasps here and there, and the looks we had been getting all evening hardened into stares. What was this? On the platform Jimmy licked his lips. He was enjoying himself in anticipation of further revelations. Jimmy Duncanson and I had gone through Trinity College together, and because he had been in agriculture, there was a common bond between us. We were more or less on the same theological wavelength; we were both married with a family; we normally sat together at lectures and had endured many a weary hour side by side, both doodling on our note-pads when the lectures were especially dry . . . and now the blighter was spilling the beans on his closest friend!

'Yes – with the police,' he repeated. 'John Stevens, your

be on our best behaviour, but I had already disgraced myself. In front of me was a plate of huge meringues, a delicacy I love; I had picked one up, bitten into it, and it had more or less exploded on my face, covering me from ear to ear in a sticky mess . . . a plastered minister!

The night before, in all the solemnity of a Presbyterian ordination, I had taken my vows in the hush of Moorton's lovely old kirk . . . a service whose atmosphere lives with me to this day. But the following night was for socializing, for presentations to various people who had helped during the short vacancy, and for a mutual 'getting to know you' by the minister, his lady and the congregation of Moorton. It was also a time for revelations about the Camerons by their friends, and words of advice from senior colleagues.

'You will find your new minister a grand preacher' (praise I certainly didn't deserve), said the Rev. Andrew Eastham, the Interim Moderator or acting minister during the vacancy.

'He's up-to-date, modern, but not too way out, not like the man who was always trying new gimmicks to get his congregation's attention. One Sunday he instructed the Beadle to be up in the church loft at the sermon, and when the text was announced, to throw down one of the pigeons which roosted there. The preacher announced his text: "Oh for the wings of a dove and I would fly away and be at rest" . . . but nothing happened. So he repeated it, twice, the second time bellowing out the words. At last the trapdoor opened and the Beadle's face appeared.

'"Minister!" he shouted, "the cat's been up and ate the doos! Wull I throw doon the cat?"' (Loud laughter.)

Andrew went on: 'He's not a blood-and-thunder preacher either, like the man who every week pounded the book-board and gave his people what for. One Sunday he was preaching on "The Day of Judgement". "There shall be wailing and gnashing of teeth," he thundered, when from be President of the Woman's Guild, President of the Mothers' Circle, and to take over as Girl Guide Captain. It seemed the Mothers' Circle were in dire straits, for 'the President has a wee boy now, and you can't expect her to carry on'! I had decided to put my foot down right at the start, and pointed out that my wife had *four* wee boys to look after, that she would do her share in church life, but one organization at a time. I don't know if I was too popular, but I was determined to clarify things right from the beginning, and hit this curious notion that many folks have – that because she is the Lady of the Manse, it is somehow the duty of the minister's wife to do everything that is asked of her.

George then went on to give me some advice. 'Despite what some folks think about ministers only working on a Sunday, you will find the ministry every bit as demanding as your vet life. You must learn to take a day off . . . go fishing, or take up golf. That's a good way to get you out, away from your parish, and rid yourself of a lot of frustration. You will no doubt find one of your Elders who will take you with him to a golf course. When I was a young minister, I used to play with my senior Elder, who, although well up in years, was almost a scratch golfer. I was just a beginner, and as the Elder won every hole I got more and more discouraged and embarrassed. To cheer me up with his way of it, the old man said to me, "Never mind, Mr Meek, one day you will have the burying of me." That was no help, for I pointed out to him that even then it would be his hole!'

George paused to let the laughter die down, then went on, 'Mind you, you've got to be careful golf doesn't get a hold on you. A certain minister's manse was right beside a fine golf course, he was a keen golfer, and one glorious summer Sunday he was up early and went out to have a look at the course. It was deserted, and he was sorely tempted to have a few holes before anybody was about. He was tempted and he fell!

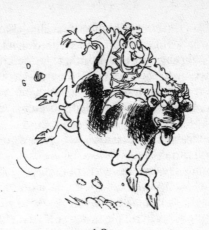

18

A World of their Own

'Is it all right for you, John, if I pick you up about seven tonight, and you can maybe take me round some of your district?' I asked on the phone.

'Fine, man,' replied John. He had been in farming and we had mutual acquaintances, so there was no reticence or reserve between us as can exist (indeed often has to exist) between a minister and his people, for a variety of good reasons. But from past knowledge, John and I were free and easy together. I was gradually getting to know my flock, being conducted by each Elder in turn and introduced to his complement of maybe twenty to twenty-five families. John was Elder in the Waterfoot area of Moorton.

'I'll take you to so-and-so' – John reeled off a few names – 'and we'll end at Low Blackpark. Man, be prepared for a shock; you never saw anything like that. They live in a world of their own out there – prehistoric!' He rang off, chuckling.

a perfect Western set. I looked carefully but could not spot any guns – but I had been warned to expect anything, so you never knew. After all, this was the family to which Basil belonged, a cousin of the present lot. Everybody knew Basil. He was none too clean, generally had a drip at the end of his nose, and was only ninety per cent or maybe less, as the local saying had it. He attended a tiny independent chapel near one of the other Tucker farms, and on one occasion was out with the pastor for a day's shooting. Suddenly Basil's 12-bore blasted off, the shot so 'adjacent' to his companion that the latter leapt heavenwards like a startled grouse.

'What – what did you do that for, Basil?' he demanded.

Basil didn't believe in using two words if one would do, and merely grunted 'Magpie – bad luck!'

'But your shot wasn't anywhere near it,' said the petrified parson.

'No matter; fire anywhere breaks the bad luck,' explained Basil patiently.

'Well, look here, don't do that again, for you nearly blew me away.'

I knew Basil quite well. He was a friendly soul, but was the plaything of anyone who wanted a laugh, on the receiving end of much hurtful hilarity, and the butt of many a hundred per cent, consciously superior mind. Yet he had a grasp of life's basic realities and was happy with what little he had. Despite the innate superstition of many country folk he had still a real piety, a sincere if simple faith, and a heart of love for all mankind as big as his large, craggy frame. I also knew cousin Donald, who was a different kettle of fish – a rogue of the first degree who would have cheated his granny, and who did cheat many, but generally managed to steer clear of the law. He was, physically, all angles; a lean individual with sloping shoulders, long arms, and a nose and chin which seemed almost to meet. He never smiled, and communicated with snorts, grunts and sly looks. He kept sheep, anybody's my size 11 wellington boots. I had my own 'Colts' plainly visible, belted over my long black waterproof coat and carried high on the hips for instant action, each gun loaded with twenty shots – in one, avian tuberculin, and in the other, mammalian. I had come to do the annual tuberculin test.

'I'm Mr Cameron, the new vet; you know, the Major's partner.'

'Us knows,' grunted one, while they continued to stare in an offhand fashion.

There followed a long pause. The conversation was distinctly languishing, so I ventured, 'Nice day!'

'Aar!' said the previous speaker, evidently the talkative Tucker.

'Ar – I mean er – can we make a start? We've quite a few beasts to do.'

'Reckon us'd best wait till vather comes,' said the speaker of the house.

Now I'm by nature a friendly soul, but what with females disappearing as soon as I hove in sight, and four males who had yet to open their mouths, though they continued to scrutinize me closely, I found it all a bit unnerving. I felt it only wanted Basil to appear waving a gun to send me scuttling for the car, but I tried again.

'I don't think we've met; I'm Cameron –'

I was interrupted. 'So ee jus' zaid,' confirmed the spokesman. He was sharp!

'Yes, but I haven't met any of you. Who's the oldest?'

The brother who talked was about seventeen, and he introduced himself as Kingsley; he nodded towards the others, who were respectively Ivan, Bernard, Cyril and baby Arthur, aged about fourteen.

'Do ee like it here, en?' asked Kingsley, providing a positive rush of conversation.

'Love it,' I said.

for the new vet. Now I am no braver than the next man, and have my own particular fears and phobias, but fear of bulls is not one of them. Respect for them, yes; care in handling, by all means; but not fear. Besides, having dealt with Ayrshire bulls, the most treacherous of any breed, I had found the Ruby Reds, as the North Devon breed was called locally, docile big creatures up till now.

'One of you come in with me, and stand behind me till I inject him, then when I grab his ring, get that ear number.'

So, accompanied by Kingsley, I braved the bull in his loose-box, gently rubbed his back, and then with a couple of quick jabs had the tuberculin in his neck. I was conscious when I rejoined the others that I had clearly passed some kind of test. It was only later, much later, that I learnt that my nice quiet beast had more than once had a go at a Tucker, and generally they approached him with pitchforks at the ready.

'Where now?' I asked.

'The yiffers and steers, us reckons,' said Cyril, finding tongue.

I was conducted to a smallish shed, which housed the 'yiffers' and steers. Never before had I seen anything like it – a world of their own indeed, for in that confined space some thirty-five to forty young beasts were milling around, treading in what had once been straw bedding but was now many feet deep, indeed half-way up to the roof. It was impossible for me to stand erect in places. There was no ring, stanchion, crush or any other means of restraint such as all the best veterinary books describe. But the Tuckers had their method, and it was sheer mayhem. I noticed 'vather' wisely retire outside, and all of a sudden we were at a rodeo. Keystones Farm, I thought, was well named, for never outside the silver screen had I seen anything quite so like the Keystone Cops as what followed now. Here we were, right back to the slapstick, custard-pie days, though when I the other grasping its nostrils, and with a heave, as I had often seen my old boss in Scotland do, I threw it to the ground, put a knee on its jaw and jabbed in approximately the approved areas – when lo! there was a great calm. It was just as if, in the middle of the aforementioned saloon fight, somebody had suddenly said, 'Whoa, there!', or the James brothers had walked in, and everybody paused, chairs ready to crash on an opponent's skull, fists drawn back for the right uppercut, or bottle about to be hurled at the large mirror which all good saloons seem to require – presumably so that a bottle can be thrown at it. It was something like that, and I was suddenly conscious that the whooping had ceased and I was being closely scrutinized by five pairs of eyes.

'Darn me, but Oi nivver saw that done before,' said Kingsley. 'How was it you did it?'

So I showed them again, picking the smallest animal I could see, and in that moment I knew I was accepted as an equal, a true, fully-paid-up member of the Tucker brotherhood. From henceforward over the years our relationship was grand. I could say anything to them and they would take it, and by golly they said plenty to me in return. They could speak, all right!

I don't know how long it took me to test those few bullocks – a whole morning easily, when normally, with animals properly housed and restrained, I would reckon to get through around 200. I only know that eventually the torture was over. I fought my way through the steaming mass of bodies, human and bovine, all covered in dung, ninety per cent proof, and reached fresh air and father, who surveyed us as we came out, uttering a few expressive 'aars' and 'uurs'. I was absolutely limp and glad to avail myself of the offer of a wash in the house, having first divested myself of my once black, now greenish-brown, coat, and scrubbed my wellingtons. Various maidens fled before me as I was postman friend had gone one cold winter day to deliver the Keystones mail, and had been astonished to find the front door open and a tree trunk sticking out of the doorway. He followed it in over the stone floor of the living-room, and found to his amazement that the other end of the tree was actually blazing in the enormous, ancient fireplace; every so often some muscular Tuckers would slide it in a bit further, all to save them sawing it up. I dare say they managed to get the door shut by night.

The odd thing was that the Tuckers seemed to prosper. They never seemed in a hurry, but, apart from gymkhanas locally, they had little interest outside their work. I don't know if the sons were paid wages or simply given their keep, but 'vor zurtain zure' they made money, acquired more land, and even bought a town house, where the young ones occasionally lived, and had to acquire two television sets because they could seldom agree on which programme to watch. For a time they broke out into a positive rash of spending, and reminded me of a story currently going the rounds of a farmer who came in from Exmoor and plonked a biscuit tin on the bank counter, instructing the teller to check it, for there was, he said, £1,000 there. The teller unfolded the crumpled mass, laboriously ploughed his way through it and said, 'Nine hundred and ninety-nine pounds, sir.' The farmer maintained there was £1,000 and insisted it be recounted. Still it came to £999, whereupon the farmer's wife said, 'Dang me, 'Erb, us's brought the wrong tin.' Thus the Tuckers – wild, untameable, unpredictable, rough and ready, yet intensely loyal to their friends, sympathetic to anyone in need. I suppose that they were the stuff that the old pioneering families were made of, and they had the same piety and godliness, despite their rough ways. This was not a natural thing for them, but acquired from mother, who, quite late in life, had found a real, personal faith, an anchor to hold her in life's storms, and longed that each of her

The car swung into the yard, a typical old-style Ayrshire steading with the house forming one end and the farm buildings two sides of a square, of which the entrance was the fourth part of the square.

'Look in there,' said John, clutching my sleeve. 'Leave your lights on!'

I obeyed and beheld a most ancient Morris with canvas hood, and beside it a large, modern Rover. On both, hens were roosting.

'John drove that old car for near thirty years,' I was informed. 'He would just chase the hens oot, gie the seat a bit dicht wi' his sleeve, an' away to the market. He's only had the Rover about a year an' he's been in the ditch wi' it three times already, blind drunk, but aye blaming it on this new-fangled machine. I think the auld car kent its way hame by itsel'.'

This, then, was my background knowledge of the Baird brothers, who, as John the Elder had predicted, were indeed sitting on either side of the fire, with their feet up and their pipes drawing nicely. I only got one glimpse of their amazing prowess at unfailingly hitting the target from a great distance as they spat towards the fire, but on the strength of that one demonstration I should say Davie, the older brother, was the champion – after all, he'd been longer at it!

John introduced me as the new minister, and they received me with courtesy and gravity, ushering me to a chair. All the chairs were ancient straight-back wooden models. I looked surreptitiously around me, and John Baird's eyes spotted my glance alighting on the table.

'My grandfather made that,' he announced. Sure enough, there was one leg very much thinner than the rest, with a cat even at that moment sharpening its claws on it. The room was bare, carpetless, with of course a stone floor. The fireplace was ancient, enormous, like many I had seen in Devon when first I went there. Beside the fireplace sat a huge could tell me the 'heads of the sermon' that James Black had once preached.

'Man,' he said, 'in these days the preacher took you by the scruff of the neck and dangled you over the pit o' hell, till you could smell your clathes singein' and decided you would do onythin' to get oot o' landin' there.'

I was mightily impressed by this armchair theologian. I ventured to ask if he'd been at Moorton kirk lately, and he fixed me with his eye and said, 'I've heard you.' Clearly my preaching, which some thought too evangelical, was milk and water to John Baird, compared with the 'real preachers they had long syne'.

Then John turned to his schooling in the tiny one-teacher school at Waterfoot. What an amazing 'dominie' had been there! I knew from the records that from that little country school had come two doctors, three lawyers, half-a-dozen ministers, an MP and a New Zealand Cabinet Minister – and these 'country loons' like John, who had stayed on as a farmer where his father had farmed before him, yet whose knowledge, grasp of world affairs and home spun philosophy were the fruits of seed sown by that lone schoolmaster in one tiny out-of-the-way hamlet. Now and then as he talked, John's sense of humour would shine through, and I realized for myself what others had already told me, how in the old Waterfoot discussion group he had been such a live-wire and doughty debater. But the night was drawing on . . .

'You'll put up a prayer afore ye go, meenister?' asked John.

I did, as was my wont, but after the flow of eloquence I'd heard my words seemed poor, stumbling things. So we departed for the car, with John's solemn 'Good-night to you both' speeding our departure.

'Well, what do you think?' asked John the Elder as we got into the car.

earnings augmented by a legacy from a brother who had made good overseas.

I mused long before the study fire that night on my two 'prehistoric' families. One ill-educated, ignorant even – the other well-educated, knowledgeable. The one close-knit as a family – the other fragmented. The Tuckers with their simple piety and code of living – John Baird with his considerable theological and philosophical knowledge. I thought of them long, and as I went to bed I had a picture of an old man facing the years, with only a bottle for his companion. There was no doubt in my mind which family had won, in this race of life.

'Iss that so now?' replied the shepherd. 'And how many sheep would you be haffing in your hirsel?'

'About half a million,' replied the Bishop, without batting an eyelid.

The shepherd was greatly astonished. 'Haff a million! Haff a million! Whateffer do you do at the lambing time?'

While not possessing gaiters or other clerical attire comparable to that of the Bishop, I too had my little flock at Moorton. We didn't have anything quite the equivalent of the lambing season of my vet days (a period in my former life I miss to this day); none the less, there were particular seasons in the life of one's flock and in the yearly round.

There was, for example, the Wedding Season. This tended to be split into two distinct parts: in spring, before 1 April, or early autumn. In the early days, I assumed in my innocence that spring weddings were due to the romance of that season when 'a young man's fancy lightly turns to thoughts of love'. The autumn I presumed to be a practical time of year in a farming community, when the harvest was safely gathered for another year. My sentimental notions were speedily shattered when I learnt that romance or expediency had nothing whatever to do with it. It was simply that these, then, were the times of year when maximum rebate of income tax could be reclaimed by a married man, and I was astonished to learn of a city colleague who actually married ten couples on the optimum Saturday of spring. How sadly do our dreams depart!

The Manse door-bell rang, and there, looking somewhat apprehensive, stood George Reid and Betty Thomson, with their attendants. They had come for a rehearsal of their wedding of the next day – a quite unnecessary proceeding, for we had already been through the whole service and subsequent reception festivities on several occasions. But couples, or more correctly, brides, like to savour the great a man clutching a handkerchief passed right behind the wedding group, and handed the handkerchief, with a few whispered words, to the person at the end of the pew which held the bridegroom's family . . . parents, brothers, sisters. The hankie was passed from hand to hand with the same few words of explanation, while I, somewhat curious as to this wedding version of 'pass the parcel', continued with the words of the service. Eventually the handkerchief reached the bridegroom's father, who was right at the end of the row, next to the wall, and he took the proferred hankie and casually put it to his mouth. His teeth had arrived! Judging by his slick, wristy action, I would say it was not the first time he had carried out this public procedure with his molars, managing somehow, with splendid camouflage, to get them right way up in his mouth.

We came to the vows.

'Do you, George, take this woman, Betty, to be your wedded wife, and do you promise to be to her a loving, faithful and dutiful husband till God shall separate you by death?'

George thought a moment while I peered at him and nodded, indicating that his turn had come. I thought I'd need to kick him, but finally he nodded and murmured, 'I do.'

'Do you, Betty, take this man George to be your wedded husband . . .'

I paused to take a breath, and the bride immediately, cheerfully, chirruped, 'I do.'

I completed my question, and the girl again made her affirmation, surely making clear to her bemused bridegroom her undying fealty! But the look he gave her tended to suggest, 'Trust you to use four words when two would do!'

Then came the moment for the couple to kneel in that most lovely part of the service where the Aaronic blessing, to time. Our present caller peered up at me from beneath a downcast countenance, and asked, 'Are you the minister . . . him that was the vet?'

What difference the vet title made, I'm not clear, unless the caller thought vet-ministers had more ready cash than ordinary ones, but I acknowledged I was the minister.

'Well, you see, Father . . . er, Reverend . . . I've been walking frae Liverpool wi' just some lifts, to get tae Glesca' tae see ma auld mither. She's in a gey bad way, and I wondered if you could help me.'

I pondered a moment. He was probably an old rascal and I was a ready 'touch', but maybe, just maybe, his story was true; Glasgow was not far away, and we were, as Christians, to 'be not forgetful to entertain strangers unawares'.

'I dare say we can manage a bus fare,' I responded, handing over half-a-crown.

'You widna' hae a cup o' tea? I hivna ett since yesterday.'

'Come in and we'll give you something.'

'That's rale kind o' ye.'

Janet gave him bacon and eggs, while the boys looked on with big eyes and the dog with suspicious ones. He told us his name was Willie McCafferty . . . told us again that his mother was very poorly and not expected to last long . . . confessed, as he leaned back in the chair picking his teeth, that he had not been a very good son, and had not seen his old mother for five years . . . recounted, almost with tears, what a mess he had made of his life but would like to make a fresh start, and could I give him a book to help him? Much moved, I gave him one of Professor Barclay's books of daily Bible studies, and another half-crown, and eventually he left.

A month later he called again, wondering if I could help him with something as he was on his way to Birmingham to look for work.

'How's your mother?' I asked.

but eventually there was a stirring in the corner. Now, there had been a couple of burglaries in the parish in the past week, and, convinced I was facing a desperado, I kept my distance and shouted, 'Come out of there! Don't you dare move!'

How he was to do this (I had now ascertained the 'body' was male) he clearly didn't know, so compromised by sitting up on the pile of logs where he had been lying. In the light of the torch, I recognized Willie McCafferty. He seemed placid enough, and so, feeling somewhat sheepish at my over-reaction, I invited him into the house.

'What were you doing in there?' I asked sternly.

'Och, I came to see if you could help me, but when there was naebody in, I just went for a sleep till you came back.'

Feeling sorry for the poor shauchly creature now, I put the kettle on to give him a cup of tea, which he had just started when the village constable, plus a colleague from the neigh-bouring town, burst on the scene, demanding, 'Have you got him?'

'I've got him, Jimmy, but I think maybe I've wasted your time. He's a tramp kind of body called Willie McCafferty, and he's been here before, but when I stepped on him in the pitch black of the coal-house, I have to admit I got a fright.'

'He'll likely be the burglar,' said the policeman, coming with his colleague into the kitchen where sat our wanderer.

'What's your name?' demanded P C McCluskey.

'Hugh Murphy,' replied our 'guest'. I gaped!

'What were you doing here?' shouted the bobby. I thought he was about as excited as I was, but I suppose if you have had two robberies in a week in a district where a forgotten dog-licence is about the only regular crime, you might be excused for getting a bit uptight.

The tramp protested that he had been doing nothing, only waiting to see the minister.

'Some story!' snorted the officer of the law.

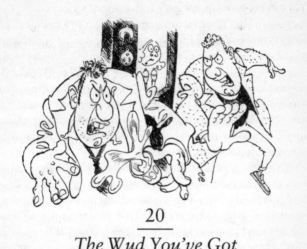

20

The Wud You've Got

In my early months as a minister I spent long hours in the study, not only preparing for meetings, Sunday School, Bible Class, Youth Fellowship and the Sunday sermons, but just thinking, planning, and examining my ministry. Early on I came to the conclusion – which has remained with me – that I was not a committee type of man. I could cope with the Sunday congregations, I loved visiting people, young, middle-aged and old, in their homes, but when it came to Session meetings and the like, I was uptight beforehand and drained afterwards. I was abundantly blessed in my wife in a host of ways, and on committee nights she was a tower of strength with her quiet support and understanding.

I came out of a Kirk Session meeting one night early in my stay at Moorton very upset. Things had not gone well. Elders had argued, decisions had been deferred, work I wanted to see begun had not been agreed upon – in short I felt it was a mess. As we left the meeting-room, Duncan the was my own Elder, Jimmy Rodgerson, quiet, understanding, loyal, true. My thoughts turned to my two golfing partners, Tom McMichael, a retired policeman, and Ian Bryce, the local vet and a good friend. Then there were farmers like Jimmy Gibson with his quaint, old-fashioned ways and pawky sense of humour . . . Jim Shankland and Jim Grant, who were great practical helps, and ploughed and worked the enormous Manse garden every year.

As I thought round them all, and many others, I came to the conclusion that I was really a lucky man in my office-bearers, and maybe my dissatisfaction at times was entirely my own fault in trying to rush change. Andrew Eastham had said to me, 'Always remember . . . quick in the town, but slow in the country. Take your folk along with you and hasten slowly.'

I concluded that night that he was right – that there wasn't much wrong with the wood, only with the man trying to work it, and I should leave things to evolve slowly and just do my weekly work. For there was plenty of that, as varied as ever my vet's life had been.

'Mr Cameron! Can you come right away?' said the agitated voice on the telephone. 'Mrs McMinn has tried to commit suicide in the butcher's shop.'

The oddest thought came into my mind . . . 'What an appropriate place for the deed!', but aloud I replied, 'I'm on my way.'

We had no resident doctor in the village and most of the men were away at work, so I imagine they felt a vet-minister was the best person available. I had visited the McMinn home twice. They were the poorest family in the parish, and although they had never been in a church in their lives, I tried to visit every home in the district. The first time I called, they were breaking up the sideboard to fuel the fire, because they had no coal. The second time, the house was in darkness and over the years, but once during the night the building was broken into and our Property Fund box, which had little in it, stolen. He must have been a clean thief because he had then proceeded to wash his hands in the vestry wash-hand basin.)

My young visitor just wanted to do what many have done: call for higher help in a domestic situation that had got beyond him. He came again – and again – and I like to think that he at least found peace there. I was reminded of the old man who used to go into a large city church every day and just sit there. One day the minister asked him what he did each day. The old man smiled and said, 'I look at Him, and He looks at me.'

That's real prayer!

'You've got a visitor,' my wife informed me when I came home at tea-time from a round of visits. 'He's been here for two hours.' The poor girl had been plying him with cups of coffee and conversation until my return.

He proved to be an alcoholic called Jim, who had just happened to get off the bus at Moorton, he didn't really know why, and had made his way to the Manse to look for help. He didn't want money, simply somebody who could maybe help with his wasted life. For it was wasted: he was jobless; his marriage had broken up; he had a wife and four children somewhere who couldn't put up with his drinking any longer. He had a prison record for violence, had been 'dried out' innumerable times in mental hospitals, and was now a broken, beaten wreck of a human being, scarcely able to eat, only drink – even meths. He had been employed in the family business of monumental sculptors, and had served in the war with distinction, becoming a sergeant-major, but after years of sponging off his parents he had finally been thrown out of the business. Now he was a wanderer – a poor ruin of what had been an intelligent man, a skilled worker over the years, usually with little success, and the tragedy is that many of them deep down are very likeable people. But it has coloured my thinking ... and actions. I accept that many finer Christians than me enjoy a drink, and in no way do I stand in judgement on folks who like a glass with friends and can control their drinking. Often I've been misunderstood, laughed at or downright condemned because I don't drink ... but Jim and his like, and a string of broken marriages caused by the bottle, always come to mind ... I feel – who knows? – that maybe I or some youngster watching me at a wedding or other social occasion could become another Jim ... and I've always felt, with deep compassion for these poor souls, 'There but for the grace of God go I.'

I was given an extra task for six months – to be chaplain to a large geriatric hospital some distance away, until another man nearer at hand could be appointed. I visited every week, moving amongst the beds of old folk, some completely helpless, some just weak and weary, some mindless. On Sunday evenings some of the choir and Youth Fellowship would come with me and we would take a little service in two of the wards.

One day when I was visiting I came across a new patient, much fitter than most.

'How are you?' I asked.

'Fine, thank you, who are you?' she replied.

'I'm the chaplain.'

'But *who* are you?'

'Oh, my name's Cameron and I'm from Moorton.'

'Hah! so you're Cameron! I've no time for you,' she went on in a very correct, indeed very affected, voice.

Now I don't like affectation, and while I'd often had my leg pulled about being a vet-turned-minister and suspected that must be the reason for this madam's condemnation of claimed to me with shining eyes, '*He* was here – *He* really was!'

An unforgettable experience of – as our fathers called it – 'the Real Presence'.

'I hear you're a minister now,' said Leslie in the train one day. I replied that was so.

'Man, I thought you had more sense!' he said. 'A quarter of a vet's salary, nothing but criticism, and tell me, what good has Christianity ever done for the world?'

Leslie had been at school with me; he was brainy, and was now a lecturer at university. We had a rare old discussion, for there's nothing I like better than getting the jacket off, so to speak, and getting down to basics. I told him that the first hospital of which there was any record, the first home for the blind, the first free dispensary, had all been founded by Christians . . . surely that was some good Christianity had done in the world? I might have told him, though only thought of it afterwards, that in various ways the work of caring was still going on. I should have told him about our 'battle' and my honourable scars.

The week before had been Christian Aid week and with ten others, ministers and priests, of varying ages, shapes and sizes, I had taken the field to play against the Stirlingshire Police at football. They seemed giants compared with our little shaughly, bowly-legged team, but, feeling like Christian martyrs facing the lions, we performed in the arena, a large football field surrounded by a very big crowd carrying banners saying 'Come away the clergy' and cheering our every effort. I don't know if they were pro-Christian – but they were certainly anti-polis! My first encounter with the police centre-half knocked me half-way across the park, and it looked as if we would be slaughtered. But as time went on, it was obvious we had some hidden talents. Our goalkeeper was performing heroics, though sorely troubled with his

depends on the teacher; but from that little school at
Waterfoot, as I've mentioned elsewhere, in the lifetime of
one schoolmaster came doctors, lawyers, several ministers,
an MP, and a Cabinet Minister of New Zealand. In addi-
tion, and perhaps more important, each child was taught
well, given a love of poetry, and taught to use words, so that
in later years they formed their own debating society. Farm
children, all of them, and taught by a wise teacher on their
own wavelength – like the schoolmistress in one school who
was trying to teach the doctrine of the Trinity, a mighty
difficult subject.

'Imagine, Angus,' she said to one boy, 'you have three
sheep at home. Call one Father, one Son, and one the Holy
Ghost. They are all the same, but yet all different.'

A few days later she was revising the lesson. 'How many
persons in the Trinity?' she asked.

'Twa, miss,' said Angus.

'Oh, Angus, do you not remember me telling you about
the three sheep?'

'Aye, miss, I ken, but you see the Holy Ghost chokit on a
turnip and he's deid.'

Unassailable logic, if not theologically sound!

The lesson over, on each visit I would be seen off by the
whole school with waves and cheers. Yes, I like the 'wee
schoolies'!

I had come to Tom Longmuir's farm one April day on just
a routine visit. It happened to be milking time in their dairy
herd, and as was my custom, I had a walk up the byre before
going to the house. I loved the sight and smell of the cattle,
something I miss to this day. Tom was nowhere to be seen,
but I found his teenage son busy with the milking.

'Faither's in the hay-shed,' he informed me. 'He's busy
trying to lamb a yow.'

I made my way to the hay-shed, which was divided by

'Meenister! I'm right grateful to ye,' said Tom, 'and while you're here, maybe you would take a look at a beast. She's off her grub, doon in her milk, so there's something no' richt.'

So we headed for the byre, and I had a look at his cow. I had no thermometer, but checked her pulse and respirations, which were normal. I had a listen at her rumen, the big first stomach, and though it was a bit sluggish, it was still churning over. But I was certain what her trouble was, for while up at her fore-leg taking the pulse, the smell of acetone came to me strongly.

'She's got acetonaemia, Tom, or as maybe you would say, she's stawed. You'd better get Ian Bryce out here to give her a bottle of glucose, or a shot of insulin, or whatever he uses.'

I, of course, didn't possess any of these remedies, and I was already feeling guilty at doing a fellow vet out of a job. Tom Longmuir looked at me long and earnestly, then his face broke into a big grin.

'Man, you're a handy fellow to hiv for a meenister. If you canna' cure a beast, you can aye say a wee prayer ower it!'

I smiled too, but didn't say anything; yet I thought back to the many times when, in the middle of a hard calving, and, like many vets, I'm sure, I had indeed breathed a prayer.

We finally got to the farmhouse, saw Mrs Longmuir, had a cup of tea and a chat, and then I went on my way, feeling that maybe a vet-minister had his uses. The Longmuirs, though by no means regular churchgoers, were in their pew the following Sunday. Ah well, I thought, there's many a way to get folk to the kirk!

Christmas Eve – surely the most magical, happiest night in the year! Moorton was silent under a December moon, the roofs of the little cottages glistening from the touch of frosty fingers, the windows bright with the twinkle of fairy lights.

Manse boys hopping about in excitement at this invasion. A final rousing sing around the piano, then the climax of it all ... the Watch-night service, carol-singers in jeans, wellingtons and Rangers scarves augmenting the great crowd assembled for this service with its unique atmosphere. A great peace seemed to wrap us all around as we heard again the wondrous story of the Child laid in a manger, and felt ourselves one with shepherds, wise men and angels as we brought our worship; at midnight we sang that loveliest of all carols, 'Still the Night'.

Only one night in the life of our little community, but a night of nights, when hope was abroad in the world and in every heart the feeling of goodwill to all men, because of the One who came to bring His peace to every longing soul.

There was one man in our little community I visited every week – Davie. His wife helped at the Manse one morning a week, and when I ran her home I would stay and have a chat with Davie. We both cherished these talks. He had few visitors, and was pleased to see me, and I always learned something from this good, God-fearing man.

Davie had been a shepherd, and a good one, but long before retiring age he had to give up his work because of a bad heart. His flock was now composed of statuettes of sheep on the mantelpiece, photographs of prize tups he had bred and a few hens which his faithful collie had to content himself now by rounding up. He made crooks as a hobby, and I will always cherish the two he gave Janet and me just before he died. For Davie has come down from his last hill, and gone home to the great sheepfold where all kinds of breeds gather at the last.

I will always remember these talks we had, and in particular one story he told me. As a young lad he was apprenticed to an older shepherd up in the hills of Ayrshire. One night there was a tremendous blizzard of snow, and the old man

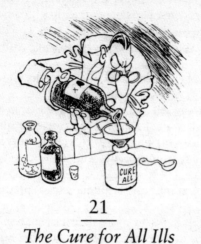

21

The Cure for All Ills

Going back to the vet world, written on the heart (or at least on a bit of paper) of every vet's wife, housekeeper, receptionist or anyone entrusted with the taking of a message is a list marked 'Very Urgent', 'Urgent' or 'Can Wait'. While it is almost certain that in the minds of all animal owners each case comes into the 'Very Urgent' category, in fact there are comparatively few which can truthfully be so described. Bloat, choke, staggers, some calvings, lambings, foalings, farrowings, etc., and the list is almost exhausted. But there is one other condition which may well appear, and indeed, be ringed around. It is known by a variety of names – urticaria, hives, blaines or nettle rash, and it is listed as 'Very Urgent' for a different reason.

'If ever you are called to a case of urticaria,' said our old Prof., 'drive like blazes or the beast will be better before you get there!'

The symptoms of this condition, particularly in cattle, can

down,' I thought, gave the thermometer a vigorous shake, and still one minute later came up with 105°. Cows with urticaria had a normal temperature. Taking the pulse up at the radial artery of the fore-leg, I was able to kill two birds with one stone, for at the same time I could count her respirations. Pulse was 80 (normal is around 50), while her respirations at 30 were about twice as fast as normal. There was something more than urticaria here. I looked at her – 'Always study the way a beast looks and the expression on its face,' the voice of old Geordie Dykes, our Professor, came back to me. We had thought it amusing then, even ridiculous, as my medical friends do yet, but I had found old Geordie knew more than we gave him credit for; perhaps we used to be a bit put off because every lecture was sprinkled liberally with his experiences in the trenches in the First World War. Yes, this cow looked ill. She had an anxious expression, maybe. The normal urticaria expression is embarrassment, like a woman being caught with her curlers in at tea-time!

The Hockings, Senior and Junior, were studying me as I studied their cow.

'Us hasn't changed our veedin', like; only thing I can think is it was the red drink.'

'Red drink?' I pounced. 'Why did you give her that, and when?'

Veterinary diagnosis is a bit like a jigsaw, putting together the pieces that you can pick up from patient and owner till all fits, or even like a detective drawing clues from unwilling witnesses. Sherlock Holmes, if he hadn't been so taken up with his wretched fiddle, could have been a first-class vet, as a lucrative sideline from his other work!

'Us drenched hur last night for she was dowie, like, off her grub, an' hur milk was down.'

'Well, ten to one your red drink caused the urticaria – something in it she was allergic to. I'll give her a jag which

'See?' said the old man, 'didn't I tell ee?' He spat elo-
quently. 'But read on – go on,' he urged. So I obliged, and
read aloud the quote from Mr A.G. of Wiltshire who'd used
the drink for thirty years and never needed a vet (probably
he kept hens, I thought). Mr W.C. (that at least was appropriate) from Berkshire declared that his father and grandfather had never been without it. My mind boggled at what
three-quarters of a pound of Epsom salts would do for
father and grandfather, but assumed it meant their stock.

'They can't all be wrong,' said the old boy, poking me in
the chest.

'Cures sunstroke – also excellent for frostbite,' I muttered.

'What's that? Speak up!' said old man Hocking.

''Twas nothing; I was only recalling a cartoon I saw
once,' I assured him. 'Look, Mr Hocking, look what your
red drink has done here. If Derek hadn't phoned me, you'd
probably have given her another dose, and that would have
killed her – one way or another.' The alternative methods
were messy even to imagine! 'If you want to have a stomach
mixture or a laxative by you, for that's all your drink is, O K
– or, better still, come to my surgery and I'll give you some
powder at half the price; but if *you* had pneumonia, would
you take Epsom salts to cure it?'

I'd said more than enough about the folly of trusting in
patent medicines and using them indiscriminately, yet I
knew almost every farmer in my practice bought these by the
dozen from the purveyors of quack remedies. Faith, I
thought, is a fine thing – but blind faith can sometimes be
utter folly.

As I drove on to my next case I recalled my old boss, who
had made up his own stomach mixture for cattle, called it
'1001' and sold it in considerable quantities. It was an
excellent prescription, and as an assistant it was some time
before he let me make up any of the mixture, indeed he

didn't need a vet, and forthwith sold him a couple of dozen 'bloat cures' and instructed the farmer to pour one over the cow's throat. This, he maintained, would scatter the gas and all would be well. Who needs vets? Some hours later I got a panic call – a re-direction from my wife from one farm to go at once to the other, for 'the beast was like to burst'. Well trained as she was, she had told them to try to keep the cow on the move and not to allow it to lie down, or very likely it would burst. (In fact the condition must be absolute agony for the beast, as the gas builds up in the rumen, or first of the cow's four stomachs, and eventually the stomach wall does, like a punctured balloon, burst. Mercifully, the pressure through the abdominal wall has usually caused such interference with breathing and the heart circulation that the animal may be unconscious or dead before the explosion.)

In the case in question, I was just in time. I had to 'stick' the cow immediately, pushing a trocar and cannula right through the stomach wall. The trocar is a sharp-pointed stilette which fits closely inside a hollow tube (the cannula), and once the poor beast has been stabbed and the trocar removed, the gas comes bubbling out of the cannula. Needless to say, this is only done when deemed absolutely necessary, and, barbaric though it sounds, the instant relief to the cow is immense. I then rounded on the farmer and, good client or not, asked him what he had been playing at, what had kept him, and a few other things beside. He was a decent sort, a good, and be it noted, an intelligent farmer, yet he had believed the bloat cure would do all, since John Pusey said so.

By now I was calming down a bit, so I grinned at him and said, 'Put not your trust in princes, even if called John Pusey.' Had to get in a dig! 'Now let's see, Mr Zeale, if we can find what caused that gas to form.'

'Reckon it was just the young clover,' said Mr Zeale.

told him he needed no vet. That cow, John, is going about this morning with a hole in its side and it's very lucky to be going about at all. We've been good clients to you and your firm in the past, man, and you have your job to do, but John, if you ever try to do mine again and advise on individual cases, so help me your headquarters will hear about it!'

Before I hung up, he managed to say he was sorry and it wouldn't happen again. My family, I hope, would agree that the old man isn't often roused, but when he is, it's like the summer storm, soon past – at least I like to think so!

But this one was not to pass so soon, for within days I was on a farm out on the fringes of the moor investigating the deaths of lambs. I did a post-mortem on two – typical cases of pulpy kidney.

'How many have you lost?' I asked the young farmer, who was a very new client and not yet well known to me.

'Reckon about two dozen,' he said. 'Yus, someways about a dozen before we asks Mr Pusey to look in, and 'bout the same since.'

'Mr Pusey?' I questioned. 'He was here – because you asked him?'

'That's right. Folks reckon he knows more about sheep than any vet'nary,' the young fellow replied rather hesitantly.

'And why have you not called him again? I expect he gave you something.'

'Oh, aye, he cuts open the lambs, bit like you, likes, only he was quicker maybe, said it was worms and gave us stuff to dose them all. He said that would do the trick.' He looked up aggressively. 'But missus reckoned we ought to give you a chance.'

I ought to have been grateful to 'the missus' for her consideration, but felt one of my summer storms coming on, so swallowed hard a few times and said, 'Look, John Pusey is not a vet. He knows a fair bit, I admit, the same way as up with same stuff you gave us last year. He really knows a lot, does Mr Pusey.'

He knows which side his bread's buttered on, I thought. He had cashed in on my work, and sold this young chap all the vaccine and serum he needed, and it was more expensive, I knew, than the brand we used! But I kept quiet. You can't win, when the Puseys of this world know all the answers and can cure all ills. In the meantime I'd written to his firm, as I'd warned him, complaining of his interference and unethical behaviour. We got a letter of apology and presumably he got a rocket, so, for a time at least, he had to walk more carefully.

Of course, this faith in a person or product is far from being confined to veterinary medicine. Give a cure-all-ills enough TV advertising, and the public is crying out for it. There is plenty of quackery about, and I find a deal of ersatz religion too. It comes in all kinds of packages, attractively labelled. There's the fellow who believes that an hour on Sunday is his weekly insurance payment to the Almighty to protect him from life's troubles, or reckons an attendance at communion and maybe Christmas is all that's needed to keep his Santa Claus kind of God happy and ensure similar Santa Claus-type benefits. I've seen dozens of this persuasion over the years. Then there's the person who has latched on to a new faith, has found in a twinkling the remedy he has long sought, and zealously seeks to bring others into his sect – for there is the truth, there alone.

I recall two instances of this at Moorton. One day two young fellows came to the Manse door, and asked if they could see the church. I showed them round, telling them something of its history. Then they came round to the real purpose of their visit. They had, some months before, become Mormons, and were now, with all the freshness and

I was well used to being put in my place and my feet set right, for each Friday in the village a meeting for children was held which sought to correct the errors of the Church as perpetuated by me and my fellow clergymen week by week. To the originator of this meeting there were few – if any – truly Christian ministers. He was a member of the Plymouth Brethren and ministers were anathema, blind leaders of the blind. Now I have a number of friends in the Brethren, and it is but right to say that not all hold this view, clergy-wise. Equally, I freely admit that a university education in Divinity does not necessarily make a Christian. If a Divinity training was a must for the practice of Christian living, then Jesus would be a non-starter, for degree He had none. I do believe, however, that to an already committed Christian, a college or university training is an aid in their future ministry. I had often chuckled over the story of the old minister who died and went to his heavenly reward, where, to his surprise, he was asked to get in the queue at the pearly gates. He was somewhat put out that he, after forty-five years of service in the one parish, should have to wait his turn – and not even a back number of *Punch* or *Country Life* to hold his interest! His chagrin turned to wrath when a stunning young blonde swept past him and was at once admitted. He demanded an explanation, to be told by the recording angel, 'That young lady passed her driving test but one week ago, but in that week she put the fear of God in more than you did in forty-five years.'

'The Fear of God' – that was the theme at the children's meetings in the village hall. I went along once or twice to show interest, but my presence was manifestly ignored. There were choruses, quizzes, sweets for prizes, all of which we had in our Sunday School. Then the twenty or so youngsters, aged from about four upwards, sat through a long address where the book was freely pounded – and a bar of chocolate given to the one who had sat most quietly. We

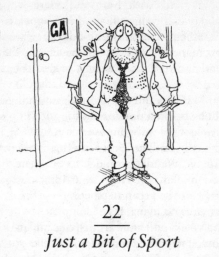

22

Just a Bit of Sport

'I hear John Pearson has got himself into trouble,' one of the Moorton Elders said to me one Sunday after morning service.

'In what way?' I asked.

'Gambling! Mind you, it's his wife and bairn I'm sorry for.'

I was sorry for Mary Pearson too, but also for John. I was also absolutely astonished. Although they lived some distance from Moorton, they belonged there originally, John was a regular in our church, and I had always thought him a steady sort of fellow, and knew he was a good husband and father. His parents were in church nearly every Sunday, and I knew they would be deeply disturbed.

So I went to visit John and Mary, and found Mary alone with their little girl in their small pre-fab house. I was shocked at Mary's appearance; she was normally a plump girl, but she had lost weight and her usually round, smiling to Glasgow tomorrow with some man to a meeting of that. I'm hoping and praying that it can help, but it seems to me it will take a miracle to save us from the awful trouble we're in . . . him and his sport.'

'Well, lass, miracles still happen. We must go on praying for one.'

And there and then we did, in simple words that came from the heart.

'Mary – don't be offended, but we have a wee fund in the church which I can use to give to anybody I think needs help. It isn't very much but it will at least keep you in food for a few weeks, and nobody but me knows who gets the money.'

So I left a little bit with the poor girl, which she promptly hid in a tin 'where John won't be able to find it'. I left her, promising to come back, and as I looked at her drawn face I felt a cold fury about the whole unholy business.

On the drive home the words 'just for sport' kept going through my mind like a chorus, and I found my thoughts drifting back to a scene from Bristacombe and my vet days.

It began when three dogs met late one evening. One was a wild, half-trained alsatian cross that came from a tinker encampment; the second was a farm collie, a well-trained, faithful animal which brought the cattle in for milking twice a day and was gentle in its handling of sheep. It slept in a barn, and could come and go as it pleased. The third was a corgi, the pet of a little girl, which had been turned out for its evening run and normally just played round about their country cottage before coming in for the night. The three dogs met up on the High Road between Bristacombe and Mortecombe, frolicked along the road together playing the canine version of 'tig', and in their joyous abandon getting further and further from their respective homes. Bye and bye they came to a field, and in that field were some interesting woolly creatures. Tired of their game, they went over the

the slaughter had taken place. The remainder of his sixty ewes were huddled together in a corner . . . stunned, shocked, terrified, exhausted after their night of terror. As we walked up the field, I spotted something white lying in the bottom corner.

'There's one you've missed, Geoff,' I said, and we headed towards it.

'It's Snowy!' exclaimed Geoff. 'She was young Billy's pet lamb last year. She's just a hogg. Poor lil' ol' thing . . . she must have been hunted into that corner and couldn't get out.'

The little hogg was far through, lying with its neck stretched out and a dreadful gash in its throat. Somehow that little hogg, trapped there by three dogs, unable to escape or fight back, brought the obscenity of the whole dirty business home to us even more than the pile of bodies. As I looked at the little animal, I realized to my complete astonishment that she was also in labour, and before our wondering eyes she gave birth to a tiny little lamb with the last of her strength. We pulled the lamb round to her head, but her eyes were already glazing in death. Yet somehow, in a strange way, this lamb from his dying hogg seemed to lift the young farmer somewhat.

'She's given us her lamb,' muttered Geoff. 'Imagine that! With her dying breath. I've never seen anything like it. You know, I think Snowy has been trying to tell me something . . . a life from the dead, in a way.'

He knelt beside the dead mother and its little lamb, already struggling to get on its feet, and as he stroked the dead little Snowy the tears flowed down his cheeks, and he kept saying over and over again, 'Dear li'l Snowy! Dear li'l Snowy!'

Then his head came up, he got to his feet, squared his shoulders and said, 'I'll struggle on – and Alex . . . I'll win through!'

chief culprit did in fact escape – no doubt to cause further killing elsewhere, when it felt like a little bit of sport.

For Geoff it was a struggle, but somehow the lesson of little Snowy had seemed a sign of hope to him. Her lamb was reared, the bank manager proved sympathetic, and Geoff fought on and won through, moving some years later to a bigger farm.

I called to see Mary Pearson from time to time, and she told me that as far as she knew John was not gambling, and that 'the meetings in Glasgow seemed to be helping'.

Then one evening John came to see me at the Manse. As I showed him into the study, he gripped my arm and said, 'Mr Cameron, you see the biggest fool in creation here – but I've learned my lesson. I haven't had a penny on a horse for three months, and it's all thanks to GA. I'd like you to come up with me to a meeting and see what they're doing up there.'

So it was arranged, and John and I drove up to the hall in Glasgow one evening where Gamblers Anonymous met in one room, the wives in another. Mary was not with us because she had their little girl to look after, and perhaps she was still a bit sceptical. I had my eyes opened that night as I saw and heard speaker after speaker tell their story. They were from every conceivable background – a company director, the manager of a large furniture shop – from well-dressed men right down to the latest recruit, who was practically in rags. He had been sleeping rough in a kind of night shelter, and pleaded with someone to go from GA to where he, and others like him, some of them also alcoholics, slept on newspapers at night. Two of the best-dressed men in GA volunteered to go to the shelter and see how they could help, and I realized that a real sense of camaraderie and caring existed between these mutual sufferers and addicts, which I found touching. All, that night, spoke of the mess they had made of their lives, and as I heard stories of

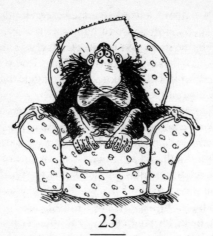

23

With Dignity and Daring

'How are you today, Mr Mackenzie?'

'I canna' complain.'

He had silicosis, making every breath an effort; he had a failing heart and kidney complications so that fluid gathered in his legs and lungs; when he wasn't in bed, he was in his chair by the fireside; he was completely limited to the four walls of a room, the outside world but a view from the window; he knew he would never be better. Yet always his reply was, 'I canna' complain' – and he meant it. It wasn't bravado, it wasn't an attempt at some kind of stoic philosophy, a shrug of the shoulders that indicated you had to just somehow put up with it all – it certainly wasn't a wish in the slightest degree to be thought gallant. He really didn't, and wouldn't complain, for he genuinely reckoned he had many blessings to count. Not an old man, he was aged far beyond his years by suffering and weakness, yet for him, his wife beside him, his family's regular visits to their dad, the glorious Technicolor. He was a Scot, really, who had gone to the States as a young man, and had now returned to his birthplace to retire. He told me of his many financial deals – about some of his clever dodges – the people in high places he knew – even his success with women: three American wives and now a Scottish one. He was able, he told me, 'to beat the hide off' anything or anyone that stood in his way. A big man physically, he was big, it seemed, no matter how he looked at himself.

'Good of you to look in, padre, but there's not a lot wrong with me, and I'm gonna ask the chief guy here to tell me straight from the shoulder just what it is, so that I can get outa this place.'

Now and then I tried to get a word in, but he kept going like a tape-recorder on his favourite theme, himself. Yes, a big man, I thought; in the phrase we had used as boys, 'a big blaw' (boaster).

'Would you like me to ask a blessing?' I inquired.

'Come again, padre?'

'Will we have a word of prayer together?' I asked hesitantly. He was amused . . . hilariously so.

'Suit yourself, padre,' he chuckled.

In prayer I felt I was talking into a void. There was no sense of a Presence here as there had been next door.

'I'll see you next week,' I said, and made my departure, glad to breathe some fresh air again.

A week went by and I saw John again. He was a little better, but greatly disturbed.

'I wish you'd see what you can do for the Yank. He's in an awfu' state, puir man!'

He was indeed. Huddled down in the bed, his large frame seemed to have shrunk and his eyes had a tortured look. He was mouthing curses at doctors, nurses, padres, his wife and the world in general. It really was a very terrible picture. It seemed he had insisted on the truth, and got it. He had

Neither did I, when I walked into his house and saw the chimp. She was huddled in an armchair by the fire, and with her outstretched arms gripping the sides of the chair and her wrinkled face resting on a cushion, she looked like a wise old grandmother watching over her family. I examined her with a sinking heart.

'I don't know what it is, Charlie, but she's dying.'

'Never! Are you sure, Alex?'

'As certain as it's ever possible to be. How long has she been like this?'

'We've noticed her getting a bit thin,' said Charlie. 'Maybe a fortnight ago we first suspected there was something, but today was the first time she just wanted to stay in her house. We brought her in here to watch her.'

The law of the wild again, I thought . . . never show weakness till it can no longer be hidden, for the weakest goes to the wall.

'Charlie, I wish I could do something, but I'm afraid it's far too late. I honestly don't know what she's got, but since monkeys are very susceptible to TB, we'll give her a big shot of streptomycin and hope for the best.'

Lulu watched me with her sad eyes as I opened my case, and scarcely moved as I injected her. She was far through, but suffering in silence, with a strange dignity about her.

She died in the night. A post-mortem showed that she had indeed tuberculosis . . . She was riddled with it, more than any animal I'd seen. Yet she had borne it with the quiet gallantry of wild things, doing at the zoo her job of making people happy and smiling, right to the end. Contact with the vet at the zoo, where she had lived till about twelve months before, revealed that they had lost many of their chimps with TB, the human strain, and the outbreak had been traced to some filthy character spitting at the animals. (Thereafter zoos found it necessary to put glass fronts on their monkey far horizons of eternity, there would still be oneness with friends on earth, and with the great Friend.

I never saw the American again. He had moved to another hospital well beyond my orbit. There was a chaplain there, I knew. I could but hope that the sick man would somehow come to terms with himself, find the peace John knew, and even in weakness be able to say, however hesitantly,

> Let me no more my comfort draw
> From my frail hold on Thee;
> In this alone rejoice with awe,
> Thy mighty grasp of me.

Drummond's *The Greatest Thing in the World*, and it set me thinking. I agreed with the famous professor about the greatest thing in the world . . . love, for I had frequently seen it in action in my ministry, and also in my life as a vet.

I recalled an incident at Hill Barton in dear old Devon. Hill Barton came about bottom of my list of favourite farms, not because of the farmer, Fred Bowden, for he was a decent young chap and good farmer, but because the farm was perched on top of a hill, and there was no road to it. You drove up a track as far as you could and then walked the rest of the way over several fields. I was re-directed by our secretary to it one day by means of a phone call to another farm I was visiting, and I had no information about the kind of animal I was to see, let alone what was wrong with it. It made life a bit difficult because I didn't know what drugs or instruments I might need, and at Hill Barton you couldn't just go out to the car and collect whatever you required — you had to trudge back over the fields to your car a long way off.

So on that bleak, cold, wet, early April day, before I left the car I checked my two cases . . . yes . . . I had most of the regular drugs and tools of the trade there. But to make sure, I stuffed the pockets of my old black waterproof coat with more bottles, draped a stomach-tube round my neck, and set off, wondering, not for the first time, who would be a vet, as the rain poured down and soon was running down my neck and stinging my eyes in the driving wind. I did some more wondering when I got near the farm and it seemed to me that half of Devon was gathered there. I suppose, to be more accurate, there were about ten people huddled on the side of a little hill just down from the farm buildings, all looking at a cow stuck in the middle of a bog. It was up to its belly in the water, and there was a rope round its horns with which the assembled company had been trying to pull it to safety. A tractor was parked nearby, with the ground at the edge of least that was the idea – but after a few yards to take up the slack of the rope, the horse also stuck. It staggered and plunged, but its feet kept slipping in the mud and the cow stayed as it was. What on earth could we try next?

Then far back in my mind a little bell tinkled, advice an old farmer had given me, yet really very obvious. I called to the young farmer to go up to the farm and bring down something. He looked at me with surprise but did as I asked, and eventually came back carrying the something, something quite small with four legs, which was giving tongue in a high-pitched voice and, since it didn't like the rain much, doing plenty of shouting. It was, of course, the cow's calf, which after the fashion of dairy herds had been removed from the mother at birth. Fred Bowden stood on the edge of the swamp holding the struggling calf . . . and almost at once the cow pricked up its ears. It gazed at the bank, and at its calf. It was then the miracle happened. The cow gave an almighty sprachle, heave and splash, and pulled itself out of that clinging, cloying muddy water. In no time it was clear, and nosing and licking its calf. We all looked on in wonderment and thankfulness. What brute force – ten men, a tractor and a horse – and scientific know-how in the shape of a vet's treatment had failed to do, love did . . . the love of a cow for its calf.

I sat back in my study chair and thought . . . that's it . . . that's my main function as a minister . . . to speak of and show a love . . . not just the love of a cow for its young . . . but a greater love, the love of God. Because it was love that sent His son into the world, to teach, to heal, to show compassion for all, yes . . . and to go the whole way to a Cross and give Himself for all mankind. Was there ever such a love, one that embraces all, good and bad, saint and sinner? And the glory of our faith – love incarnate

FOR THE BEST IN PAPERBACKS, LOOK FOR THE

In every corner of the world, on every subject under the sun, Penguin represents quality and variety – the very best in publishing today.

For complete information about books available from Penguin – including Pelicans, Puffins, Peregrines and Penguin Classics – and how to order them, write to us at the appropriate address below. Please note that for copyright reasons the selection of books varies from country to country.

In the United Kingdom: Please write to *Dept E.P., Penguin Books Ltd, Harmondsworth, Middlesex, UB7 0DA*

If you have any difficulty in obtaining a title, please send your order with the correct money, plus ten per cent for postage and packaging, to *PO Box No 11, West Drayton, Middlesex*

In the United States: Please write to *Dept BA, Penguin, 299 Murray Hill Parkway, East Rutherford, New Jersey 07073*

In Canada: Please write to *Penguin Books Canada Ltd, 2801 John Street, Markham, Ontario L3R 1B4*

In Australia: Please write to the *Marketing Department, Penguin Books Australia Ltd, P.O. Box 257, Ringwood, Victoria 3134*

In New Zealand: Please write to the *Marketing Department, Penguin Books (NZ) Ltd, Private Bag, Takapuna, Auckland 9*

In India: Please write to *Penguin Overseas Ltd, 706 Eros Apartments, 56 Nehru Place, New Delhi, 110019*

In Holland: Please write to *Penguin Books Nederland B.V., Postbus 195, NL–1380AD Weesp, Netherlands*

In Germany: Please write to *Penguin Books Ltd, Friedrichstrasse 10–12, D–6000 Frankfurt Main 1, Federal Republic of Germany*

In Spain: Please write to *Longman Penguin España, Calle San Nicolas 15, E–28013 Madrid, Spain*

In France: Please write to *Penguin Books Ltd, 39 Rue de Montmorency, F-75003, Paris, France*

In Japan: Please write to *Longman Penguin Japan Co Ltd, Yamaguchi Building, 2–12–9 Kanda Jimbocho, Chiyoda-Ku, Tokyo 101, Japan*

QUIZZES, GAMES AND PUZZLES

The Book Quiz Book   Joseph Connolly

Who was literature's performing flea . . .? Who wrote 'Live Now, Pay Later . . .'? Keats and Cartland, Balzac and Braine, Coleridge conundrums, Eliot enigmas, Tolstoy teasers . . . all in this brilliant quiz book.

The Ultimate Trivia Game Book   Maureen and Alan Hiron

If you are immersed in trivia, addicted to quiz games, endlessly nosey, then this is the book for you: over 10,000 pieces of utterly dispensable information!

The Penguin Book of Acrostic Puzzles   Albie Fiore

A book of crosswords and a book of quotations in one! Solve the clues provided, fit the letters into the grid provided and make a quotation. It's the most fun you can have with a pen and paper.

Plus five trivia quiz books:
The Royalty Game
The TV Game
The Travel Game
The Pop Game
The Business Game

Crossword Books to baffle and bewilder

Eleven Penguin Books of the *Sun* Crosswords
Eight Penguin books of the *Sunday Times* Crosswords
Seven Penguin Books of *The Times* Crosswords
and Four Jumbo Books of the *Sun* Crosswords
The First Penguin Book of *Daily Express* Crosswords
The Second Penguin Book of *Daily Express* Crosswords

Penguin Crossword Books – something for everyone, however much or little time you have on your hands.

BIOGRAPHY AND AUTOBIOGRAPHY IN PENGUIN

Jackdaw Cake   Norman Lewis

From Carmarthen to Cuba, from Enfield to Algeria, Norman Lewis brilliantly recounts his transformation from stammering schoolboy to the man Auberon Waugh called 'the greatest travel writer alive, if not the greatest since Marco Polo'.

Catherine   Maureen Dunbar

Catherine is the tragic story of a young woman who died of anorexia nervosa. Told by her mother, it includes extracts from Catherine's diary and conveys both the physical and psychological traumas suffered by anorexics.

Isak Dinesen, the Life of Karen Blixen   Judith Thurman

Myth-spinner and storyteller famous far beyond her native Denmark, Karen Blixen lived much of the Gothic strangeness of her tales. This remarkable biography paints Karen Blixen in all her sybiline beauty and magnetism, conveying the delight and terror she inspired, and the pain she suffered.

The Silent Twins   Marjorie Wallace

June and Jennifer Gibbons are twenty-three year old identical twins, who from childhood have been locked together in a strange secret bondage which made them reject the outside world. *The Silent Twins* is a real-life psychological thriller about the most fundamental question – what makes a separate, individual human being?

Backcloth   Dirk Bogarde

The final volume of Dirk Bogarde's autobiography is not about his acting years but about Dirk Bogarde the man and the people and events that have shaped his life and character. All are remembered with affection, nostalgia and characteristic perception and eloquence.